Understanding Attention Deficit Hyperactivity Disorder

Understanding Health and Sickness Series
Miriam Bloom, Ph.D.
General Editor

Understanding Attention Deficit Hyperactivity Disorder

L. Susan Buttross, MD, FAAP

University Press of Mississippi
Jackson

Publication of this book was made possible in part by the
Phil Hardin Foundation.

www.upress.state.ms.us

The University Press of Mississippi is a member of the Association of
American University Presses.

Illustrations by Wendy Eddleman

First edition 2007

∞

Library of Congress Cataloging-in-Publication Data

Buttross, L. Susan.
    Understanding attention deficit hyperactivity disorder /
L. Susan Buttross. — 1st ed.
        p. cm. — (Understanding health and sickness series)
    Includes index.
    ISBN-13: 978-1-57806-882-1 (cloth : alk. paper)
    ISBN-10: 1-57806-882-7 (cloth : alk. paper)
    ISBN-13: 978-1-57806-883-8 (pbk. : alk. paper)
    ISBN-10: 1-57806-883-5 (pbk. : alk. paper) 1. Attention-deficit
hyperactivity disorder—Popular works. I. Title.
    RJ506.H9B88   2007
    618.92'8589—dc22   2006102840

British Library Cataloging-in-Publication Data available

Contents

Acknowledgments

There are many who I wish to thank for their help and support in the development of this book. The expert reviewers included physicians Adrian Sandler, Grayson Norquist, and Valerie Arnold. The guidance from my editor and publisher were needed by this novice and greatly appreciated. Lorie Naef, a long-time friend and dedicated social worker, gave immeasurable help throughout the entire process. The Child Development Clinic staff, my second family, helped me in many ways to get this project completed—taking calls, putting up with my crowded schedule, helping me find that extra time to work, and listening to ideas about this book were part of the daily routine at the office. Two particular staff members deserve a special thanks, Ruth Willis, who helped me through all of my computer inadequacies, and Lee Ann Swartzentruber, who was a wonderful resource for finding needed information. I have the extreme pleasure of teaching residents and students, many of whom during their month-long rotation participated in one way or another in the creation of this project. Two stand out as being especially helpful, Jonny Byrnes and Mark Lee. I also thank the thousands of children and teens with ADHD and their parents who I have seen over the years. Their unique experiences enhanced my knowledge and skills to better treat others.

Finally, I must thank my wonderful family, who has always had faith in me. My children, Robin, Erin, Sarah, Tim, and Charles, all have been gifts who have allowed me to learn on the job. Their experiences no doubt have made me a better pediatrician. Last and most importantly, I must thank my best friend and husband, Robert, for his faith in me and his patience and encouragement.

Introduction

There is a huge amount of information available on attention deficit hyperactivity disorder (ADHD) in the scientific and lay literature. Just a look on the Internet reveals everything from ways to diagnose the disorder in one easy checklist to the many supposed cures that are offered. Separating fact from fiction is important, but it can be difficult when dealing with the volumes of information available.

The core symptoms of this condition, which is most commonly diagnosed in children, are inattention, hyperactivity, and impulsivity. These symptoms can occur in almost anyone at one time or another in his or her life. The broadness of these symptoms makes it tempting to put anyone with inattention or hyperactivity into the same box. Even the name ADHD is confusing. Some individuals may have profound problems with inattention and concentration but appear to sit still with no hyperactive or impulsive behavior noted. Further confounding the issue is the fact that inattention and hyperactivity can be the result of other conditions or behaviors. The old adage, "If it looks like a duck and walks like a duck, then it must be a duck," is not true when dealing with those who have the symptoms of ADHD. External forces such as social issues, classroom arrangement, and level of expectations can adversely affect a person's ability to concentrate and appropriately respond to the environment. It is no wonder that controversy remains as to what ADHD is and who really has it.

Up to 8 percent of elementary-age children in the United States are affected by ADHD, with similar numbers being reported in other countries. Furthermore, there is growing evidence that ADHD is not just a disorder of childhood, but one that often continues into adulthood. Because the numbers of affected individuals are so high, the question has been raised as to whether ADHD is a real disorder or simply a difference. Thom Hartmann, a radio host and author, suggested that historically the traits held by those with ADHD likely put them at an advantage. The ability to respond instantaneously and reflexively to prey may have made hunters more successful. In *Dreamers, Discoverers, and Dynamos*, the psychologist Lucy Jo Palladino discussed the differences that ADHD individuals possess that may put them at an advantage in some areas. In fact, numerous famous individuals are said to have had many of the traits of those with ADHD. Perhaps Benjamin Franklin, Thomas Edison, and Albert Einstein would not have been so inventive and successful had they not possessed some level of hyperactivity and impulsivity. Certainly, had Franklin thought hard about using a key and string to test out his theories of electricity, he may have realized the potential danger and never made the first attempt. Edison was known to sleep only a few hours each night, rising before dawn to work on his latest invention. Einstein was very slow to speak as a child; he was a poor student in school and often in trouble for his behavior. Could young Albert have been distracted by his many creative and inventive thoughts? Contemporary creative and successful people who have spoken openly about their life with ADHD include the political strategist James Carville, actors Vince Vaughn and Tracey Gold, Pulitzer Prize–winning columnist Clarence Page, and former quarterback Terry Bradshaw. The traits of spontaneity, impulsively quick thinking, and rapidly changing wit make them who they are.

The symptoms of ADHD have been noted in children for many years. In his book *Attention-Deficit Hyperactivity Disorder*, Larry Silver, a psychiatrist at Georgetown University, noted that Heinrich Hoffman's 1863 nursery rhyme was likely about a young boy who had ADHD:

> *"Phil, stop acting like a worm,*
> *The table is no place to squirm."*
> *Thus speaks the father to his son,*
> *severely says it, not in fun.*
> *Mother frowns and looks around,*
> *although she doesn't make a sound.*
> *But, Philipp will not take advice,*
> *he'll have his way at any price.*
> *He turns,*
> *and churns,*
> *and wiggles,*
> *and jiggles*
> *here and there on the chair.*
> *"Phil, these twists I cannot bear."*

Most historical references to ADHD describe children and their behaviors. Studies indicate, however, that some symptoms such as hyperactivity and impulsivity decrease with age, while other symptoms may persist into adulthood. Difficulties across multiple settings, including home, school, and peer relationships, typically occur. Those with undiagnosed ADHD can experience long-term negative effects on their academic performance, social relationships, and occupational achievement. Individuals with ADHD are not the only ones who are affected by their disorder; parents, teachers, siblings, peers, and coworkers may all feel the impact of untreated ADHD. Although I have diagnosed and treated ADHD for more than twenty years, I did not truly understand the far-reaching and profound impacts that this disorder can have on a family until one of my own children was diagnosed with it. Though very talented and wonderful in his own right, the symptoms of my son's ADHD sometimes have made traditional school difficult for him.

In this book, I discuss what ADHD really is, who gets it, and why. A step-by-step plan is given on what should be expected in the evaluation of someone who is suspected of having ADHD. I also describe disorders that may mimic the symptoms of ADHD. Treatment options, behavioral charts, and medications available are reviewed in depth, including the pros and cons of the various treatments. I provide behavioral charts and others tricks of the trade that will make school, home, and social life more successful. Finally, I explain how scientific studies are designed to develop reliable research in ADHD, and I summarize the latest genetic studies, the newest findings in brain differences, and novel treatments. The appendix provides contact information for general resources and support and advocacy groups, web sites, and recommended reading that will further enhance knowledge and lend support for ADHD patients and their parents and teachers.

Though we understand much about ADHD, there is still a lot to be learned. A clearer idea of what ADHD is and how this interesting disorder can be treated can make a huge difference in the lives of many who are affected. Whether ADHD is a disorder or difference, evidence suggests that with the proper understanding, acceptance, and environment, these children, teens, and adults will not only be successful but also will have a great deal to contribute to our society.

Understanding Attention Deficit Hyperactivity Disorder

1. What Is Attention Deficit Hyperactivity Disorder?

"Jason got two days detention yesterday for tapping his foot on the floor, not being able to sit still, and talking to another student during class because he forgot his pencil in his locker. I wanted to call his teacher and say, Mr. Rodgers–style, 'ADHD, can you say that?'"

—E-mail message from a frustrated mother
of a child with ADHD

Although ADHD is a documented and treatable disorder, misinformation and misdiagnosis of children and adults still exists. Many other disorders and some behaviors and learning problems can mimic ADHD. A clear understanding of what ADHD is will help to avoid inappropriate or missed diagnosis.

More than a century ago Dr. George Still presented to the Royal College of Physicians in London a paper describing the behaviors of twenty children with inattention, excessive motor activity, and poor "inhibitory volition." These children had symptoms very similar to those individuals now diagnosed with ADHD. Dr. Still later published an article entitled "Some Abnormal Psychical Conditions in Children" in which he further described these children and other behavioral issues, including discipline problems, defiance, dishonesty, and "lawlessness." These latter behaviors, which are now the separately defined behavioral disorders of oppositional defiant disorder and conduct disorder, are sometimes seen in conjunction with ADHD.

The initial descriptions of ADHD focused on the behavioral aspects, particularly hyperactivity. Even into the 1980s children with attentional problems, hyperactivity, learning disabilities, and borderline intelligence were labeled as having "minimal brain dysfunction" or "minimal brain damage." Over the last twenty years, however, a better understanding of the individual disorders has allowed further separation of learning disabilities from behavioral symptoms.

The first Diagnostic and Statistical Manual of Mental Disorders (DSM), published in 1968 by the American Psychiatric Association, labeled the condition hyperkinetic disorder of childhood. The core symptoms recognized at that time were inattention and hyperactivity. By 1980, however, the DSM-III reflected a shift in thought: inattention was the primary presenting problem and the disorder was named attention deficit disorder. Formal diagnostic criteria were developed in the 1980s, and the DSM-IV, published in 1994, further defined and clarified the diagnostic criteria that are used today.

The Symptoms of ADHD

In the DSM-IV, the American Psychiatric Association categorized the diagnostic criteria of ADHD into two major groups: inattention and hyperactivity/impulsivity. At least six symptoms of inattention or hyperactivity/impulsivity must exist in order for a child to receive the diagnosis of ADHD. These symptoms must be present for at least six months continuously and should be inconsistent with the developmental level of the child.

According to the DSM-IV, a child with inattention often:

fails to pay close attention to details or makes careless mistakes;
has difficulty in tasks that require sustained attention in play, school, or work;

does not seem to listen when spoken to;
does not follow through on instructions and tasks for
    schoolwork, chores, or work;
has difficulty organizing tasks and activities;
avoids tasks that require prolonged mental effort;
loses things easily;
is distracted by extraneous stimuli; and
is forgetful in his or her daily activities.

A child with hyperactivity/impulsivity often:

fidgets with hands or feet or squirms in his or her seat;
is up out of his or her classroom seat or in other places
    when remaining seated is expected;
runs or climbs when it is inappropriate (for teens the
    symptom may be restless behavior);
has difficulty engaging quietly in leisure activities;
is "on the go";
talks excessively;
blurts out answers before the question is complete;
has difficulty waiting his or her turn; and
interrupts or intrudes on others.

Although the name may be a bit confusing, ADHD is the
diagnostic term given whether or not the symptom of hyperactivity exists, and the disorder is now divided into three main
types:

ADHD—combined type (ADHD-CT): The symptoms
    of inattention, impulsivity, and hyperactivity occur in
    generally equal proportions.
ADHD—primarily inattentive type (ADHD-I): Inattention
    is the overriding symptom. The child is not a bother to

anyone but sits and stares out of the window or is distracted by any movement. This type seems to affect girls more often than boys but can occur in both sexes.

ADHD—primarily hyperactive type (ADHD-H): Hyperactivity and impulsivity are the overriding symptoms.

According to the DSM-IV diagnostic criteria, symptoms must be present prior to seven years of age. The reasoning behind this is that ADHD is a developmental disorder that likely has a genetic cause. Thus, the manifestation of symptoms should occur at least by the time the child enters primary school, when real demands on attention and self-control are made on the child. A bright child who works hard with a supportive and organized family may not have the ADHD-I diagnosed until after seven years of age because of the family assistance, but retrospectively, the symptoms should have been present.

The DSM-IV criteria also state that the symptoms must be continuous and present in more than one setting, such as at home, school, and work. This requirement dictates that the disorder is pervasive and not situational. If a child is only hyperactive at home, but problems do not occur in school, the hyperactivity may be behavioral or there may be inappropriate demands placed on the child at home. If the child is only inattentive in math class and not in others, then it may be a problem with math rather than ADHD or the particular teacher may have very strict behavioral expectations in the classroom.

Another important point in the criteria is that the problems should cause a significant impairment. Many individuals will have some of the symptoms described as ADHD at one time or another in their life. Some individuals are more calm and attentive than others, and the range of normal behaviors should not be so narrow that everyone is expected to behave exactly the same way. This requirement of a significant impairment is an attempt to keep the range of normal behaviors in proper perspective.

The final point used in making the diagnosis is that the symptoms must occur for more than six months continuously. ADHD is a chronic disorder and thus must be distinguished from a more transient disorder. A sudden onset of inattention and behavioral problems in a child at any age could signal a host of other issues or illnesses. Depression, illicit drug use, medications, social problems, and family discord are a few of the issues that might alter attention and behavior.

Case Example.   Cindy is a twelve-year-old in the sixth grade. She repeated the first grade and has struggled to make grades of B and C. She has never been a problematic child and actually has been described as quiet and well behaved in class. She has always had problems with completing her classroom work on time, taking timed tests, and completing homework. She has been called "not very bright" and "lazy and unmotivated" by some of her teachers. Because of poor grades, she is no longer allowed to be a cheerleader, which is something she has always loved to do. Cindy is frustrated and angry about this and says that she is trying as hard as she can. She wants help and has expressed some feelings of being "stupid." Her parents suspected that she had hearing or vision problems, due to her increasing difficulties in school, but when tested, both hearing and vision were normal.

Children with ADHD-I are often not diagnosed until an older age because of the lack of behavioral issues that usually lead to the early diagnosis of children with ADHD-H or ADHD-CT. An inattentive child may know the information when a parent studies with the child, but when required to perform in a large classroom or take a written test, the child does poorly. Scores on standardized tests given in a group setting are frequently below the child's true skill level due to the difficulty of staying on task. Expectations are lowered because of the low scores. Adequate testing by a trained psychologist or psychometrist (a person who is trained to test intelligence and academic achievement) is important for proper identification of a child with ADHD-I versus a child with a learning disability or a low intelligence quotient (IQ). A child with ADHD-I may seem to have poor reading comprehension when tested with a group, but when tested individually by a psychologist, the reading level may be normal.

Most people demonstrate signs of inattention at one time or another in their lives. Attention to detail is difficult for anyone with fatigue, illness, stress, or anxiety. In those with ADHD, however, the symptoms are present all of the time and affect life in general. Lost books, forgotten assignments, missed appointments, poor attention to details, careless mistakes, and lack of follow-through are all common complaints about those with ADHD. Children and adults with this disorder typically avoid tasks that require a sustained mental effort. Because of the inattention, reading with good comprehension is difficult. Reading for pleasure is avoided because little enjoyment is derived from the task.

The hyperactivity and impulsivity components of ADHD are more easily identified because of the commotion that is caused by these behaviors. "Driven by a motor" or "like his accelerator is stuck" are two phrases used by parents to describe their children's hyperactivity. Teacher and peer pressures may change the behaviors in older children to squirmy, fidgety behavior because being up and out of their seat is unacceptable in the classroom. School suspensions, missed recesses and field trips, and exclusion from birthday parties and other social events are common issues that these children experience. An increased rate of accidents and injuries are much more common in the child with ADHD.

Signs of impulsivity include acting and speaking without thinking about the consequence; for example, a child may consistently blurt out answers in the classroom before the question is complete. A more extreme example of impulsivity is the boy who jumped several feet from a tree when he saw his friend coming toward him. He simply forgot how high up he was. The result of that bout of impulsivity was a broken arm.

Though stories told about the severely hyperactive child are frequently comical, parents and caretakers likely do not find much humor in the disorder. Early intervention is necessary to prevent the child from harming himself, being harmed by others, or before long-term negative patterns of parenting develop. First-time parents may not recognize that their child's extreme behaviors are abnormal, and others may think that the child's behavior is the result of them being inexperienced parents. Once the child enters a structured situation, such as kindergarten, the more normal behavior of classmates makes the behavior of a child with ADHD stand out.

Case Example.   When Ross was two years old his parents had to resort to using a child harness to keep him from running off when they were in public places. At four years of age, his parents were asked to remove him from preschool due to his disruptive behaviors. His mother says that she still cannot take her eyes off of him because he will run off. She cannot count the number of times that she has lost him in a store. None of her relatives, not even the loving grandmother, is comfortable babysitting him. He has been in trouble since he entered kindergarten this year. The teachers complain that he will not complete his work and is up and out of his seat, preventing others from doing theirs. He is constantly talking and touching others and has been in "time out" numerous times due to his behavior in the cafeteria line. He dashes everywhere and loves to be the center of attention. His teachers say that Ross is not a mean child, he just cannot seem to control himself. When corrected, he will stop the behavior for a while, but then it will start right back up. The teacher recently called his mother to say that he will not be allowed to go on the next field trip because of his misbehavior.

Every aspect of a child's life is affected when severe ADHD-HI exists. If appropriate intervention does not occur early, frustration of parents and teachers may lead to inappropriate management. Such mismanagement will further confuse the issues and make it difficult to separate the true symptoms of ADHD from behavioral issues. Relationships with parents, relatives, peers, and teachers can be negatively affected in the short and long term.

Changing Symptoms

Symptoms differ depending on the age of the individual with ADHD and the severity of the disorder. In the young child, the majority of complaints center on the hyperactive and impulsive behaviors. Later in childhood and in adolescence, the problems are more focused around academics and school performance. Because the symptoms of ADHD can vary greatly, early recognition may be difficult. Although the ADHD diagnostic criteria require that the symptoms appear prior to seven years of age, the diagnosis may not be made until much later. The impulsivity and hyperactivity may not stand out greatly from the general population until the child is in a structured classroom setting. If inattention is the overriding symptom, the difficulties may become more apparent as the child moves into upper elementary school grades, when reading comprehension becomes more important. The child's social life may be affected minimally due to lesser symptoms of hyperactivity, whereas another child may have symptoms so severe that he is easily recognized as having problems in any setting. More severely affected individuals have symptoms that continue throughout their school careers. Seventy percent of those affected with ADHD will have problems that persist into adolescence. In fact, recent evidence suggests that more than 50 percent of those diagnosed with ADHD as children will continue to have problematic symptoms throughout adulthood.

ADHD in the Young Child

Toddlers are naturally active, but occasionally a child stands out far beyond what is recognized as normal. ADHD-HI is apparent in some cases as early as three or four years of age. Parents of these children frequently complain about never being able to go anywhere due to the behavioral difficulties. Shopping trips, going out to eat, or other family outings are not only difficult, they are impossible. The impulsive behaviors of these very active toddlers can put them in dangerous situations, and parents are often exhausted due to the need for constant vigilance when caring for them.

Often the parents of a child with ADHD may not recognize the behaviors as being atypical until the child enters preschool or a childcare situation and they receive complaints from the teachers and childcare workers. Disruptive behaviors that interfere with the rest of the class are common in the ADHD child. Naptime for these children is often an impossibility, and settling down to sleep at night is usually difficult. The rate for minor accidents and injuries is higher due to the impulsive nature of the child, and parents' skills are questioned by others due to their inability to control the child's behavior. Parents may make the initial visit to a pediatrician to discuss ADHD because their child has been kicked out of childcare or preschool. At this point, the stress on the family integrity can be extreme, and parents express feelings of not knowing what to do next.

ADHD in the School-Age Child

Entry into elementary school is the most common event that initiates an evaluation for ADHD. Disruptive, fidgety behavior, failure to follow directions, and incomplete work are common complaints. On the playground, these children fail to take turns and follow rules or they exhibit aggressive behaviors. The ADHD child may have to repeat kindergarten, with the reason cited as "immaturity." Unfortunately, a repeat of kindergarten alone without recognition of the disorder will do little to help the child succeed the following year.

Children with ADHD-I are not overly active; instead, there are complaints that the child is slow moving, misses instructions, loses things easily, and is never prepared. The proper diagnosis of ADHD-I is often made later in the child's school career. There may be suspicion of something being wrong as the child enters middle school, when reading comprehension becomes especially important in academic success.

ADHD in Teens

Teens with ADHD-CT or ADHD-HI will have a shift of symptoms from excessive activity to more internal and subjective feelings of restlessness and complaints of easy boredom, incomplete work, and poor grades. Although the obvious symptoms of hyperactivity and impulsivity seem to improve, the inattention can result in academic underachievement. An intelligent teen may be passed over for many opportunities because his true skill level is not recognized, leaving the teen feeling frustrated. The longer the frustration and underachievement go on, the more likely it is that the teen will develop problems with anxiety and depression. This downward spiral regularly occurs in later teen years in unrecognized, poorly understood, or untreated individuals with ADHD. Frustrated teens will often migrate to fringe groups in an attempt to fit in. The teen years are when increased drug and alcohol use occurs in an attempt to "feel better" or "fit in better."

Impulsivity is another misunderstood symptom in teens with ADHD. Social and family function and work performances are all affected by this symptom. These individuals are often viewed as rude, self-absorbed, or difficult to be around. Self reports by teens with ADHD reveal difficulty waiting in line, interrupting others, impulsive spending, difficulty driving, and an inability to inhibit emotional reactions when dealing with others. Although the hyperactivity does improve in most teens, some may continue to have problems with fidgeting, nail biting, picking at sores, and excessive talking. Appropriate treatment of these symptoms can make a major difference in the ultimate life adjustment and outcome as teens become adults.

ADHD in Adults

More than half of those diagnosed with ADHD as children will continue to have symptoms as adults. As in teens, the hyperactivity and impulsivity of the disorder evolve into more subjective feelings of restlessness and boredom. As in teens, studies have shown that adults who continue to have significant symptoms of ADHD have greater problems with accidents and injuries requiring emergency room visits and a greater number of traffic citations. Relationships and job longevity also suffer in some cases due to the impulsive nature of the adult with ADHD and the resultant problems that occur when one acts without first thinking of the consequences.

The Costs of ADHD

Though no one has ever thought of ADHD as life threatening, if left undiagnosed this disorder can result in major, life-altering events. The evidence is clear that those with untreated ADHD have poorer outcomes in academics, vocational achievement, and social adjustment and experience more legal issues when compared to their intellectual and socioeconomic peers. Early discovery and treatment of this disorder, however, can have a major impact on the ultimate outcome and well-being of individuals with ADHD.

Parents of children with ADHD are often told by others that their parenting skills are poor. The most severely affected child may develop problems as early as two-year-old preschool, when parents are asked to remove their child due to the uncontrollable disruptive behavior. That situation alone stigmatizes the child and embarrasses the family, and this first insult is usually only the first of many to come. The hyperactive child is frequently not invited to play groups or birthday parties early on because of the disruptive and impulsive behaviors. Attending church, going out to eat, or making a shopping trip with an ADHD child can turn into a nightmare for the parent. Increased stress, frustration, anxiety, and recurrent bouts of anger can all occur as parents attempt to cope with these difficult-to-manage children. When a parent has poor understanding of the disorder and inadequate coping skills, children with ADHD are at a greater risk of child abuse. Parental depression, low self-esteem, self-blame, and social isolation are often part of the negative spiral. Other problems that may occur for the parents of a child with ADHD include increased rates of employment disruption, marital problems, and alcohol and substance abuse.

Entering school presents another set of problems for the child with ADHD and his parents. Frequent calls home, time in detention, and school suspensions occur more often for the child with ADHD. Up to 50 percent of children with significant and continuous problems with ADHD have repeated a grade. As many as 30 percent of teens with ADHD will drop out or fail to complete high school as compared to 10 percent of teens without ADHD. Appropriate recognition, diagnosis, and treatment, however, have been shown to decrease the failure and dropout rate to one that is comparable to those without ADHD.

Another important issue for the ADHD child is socialization. Between the ages of five and eighteen, more hours of a child's waking life are spent at school than any other place. Most socialization is connected to school through extra-curricular activities such as cheerleading, sports, band, art, and debate. Children with ADHD can be stigmatized by their behavior. If a child is disruptive, impulsive, and hyperactive, then he may be tagged as a troublemaker, a bad sport, immature, or a class clown. If left without intervention, as children with ADHD move into their teen years they show poor participation in group activities and have fewer friends. The social isolation experienced by inadequately treated teens makes them more vulnerable to peer groups involved in illicit drug use and antisocial behaviors. The psychiatrist Joseph Biederman reported that teens who are not treated for ADHD are much more likely to have problems with substance abuse, being 78 percent more likely to be addicted to tobacco and 58 percent more likely to use illegal drugs.

There is evidence that adolescents who have struggled with untreated ADHD are more likely to have minor traffic violations, vehicular accidents, and visits to emergency rooms for injuries than those who are treated for their ADHD. In their first two years of driving, adolescents with ADHD are involved in automobile accidents more often than those without the disorder. As expected, they are more likely to be at fault and are more likely to incur injuries. The psychologist Russell Barkley found that, when compared to those without the disorder, ADHD teens reported more suspended or revoked licenses (42 vs. 28 percent), more accidents in which the car was totaled (49 vs. 16 percent), and more hit-and-run accidents (14 vs. 2 percent).

According to the 1999 "Annual Report of the Surgeon General," an astounding 9.7 million physician office visits occurred due to accidents and injuries that appeared to be associated with ADHD. In 2001 the "Physician Drug and Diagnosis Audit" reported that 30 to 50 percent of child mental health referrals were due to ADHD. The 2003 "National Survey of Children's Health Needs" found that children with ADHD have higher medical costs, an estimated $500–1300 per year higher than children without the disorder. Likewise, adults with ADHD incur an estimated $3000 of increased medical costs per year.

Ultimate academic and vocational achievements are lower in adults with untreated ADHD than in those without the disorder. Continual problems with impulsivity and inattention can affect jobs and relationships. Adults who have struggled with untreated ADHD are much more likely to complain of anxiety, depression, and physical ailments. Often, in an attempt to alleviate the feeling of anxiety and depression, there is an increase in substance abuse.

Summary

According to the DSM-IV diagnostic criteria, individuals with ADHD suffer from two major groups of symptoms: inattention and hyperactivity/impulsivity. In those individuals with ADHD-CT, the symptoms of inattention, impulsivity, and hyperactivity occur in generally equal proportions, whereas in those with ADHD-I inattention is the overriding symptom and in ADHD-H hyperactivity and impulsivity are the overriding symptoms. The symptoms differ depending on the age of the individual with ADHD and the severity of the disorder. In the young child, the majority of complaints center on the hyperactive and impulsive behaviors. Later in childhood and in adolescence, the problems are more focused around school performance. Teens and adults suffering from ADHD are more prone to physical injuries, anxiety, depression, and substance abuse, all of which have negative effects on relationships with family members, peers, and coworkers.

2. What Causes Attention Deficit Hyperactivity Disorder?

"Each day is like being at the fair . . . roller coaster rides filled with ups, downs, and loop-de-loops, with sideshows of frustration and bewilderment . . . ending with thoughts of hope for the next day. How can he be such a great kid and have so much trouble?"
—A mother speaking about her gifted son with ADHD

Up to 8 percent of elementary school children in the United States are affected by ADHD, a condition characterized by developmentally inappropriate inattention, hyperactivity, and impulsivity. ADHD is not unique to this country, however. Studies from fifteen countries on five continents have reported the condition, with prevalence ranging from 1 to 20 percent across these countries. Although this range may seem broad, social expectations, genetics, environment, diagnostic criteria, and teaching styles may have bearings on the numbers. There are no significant racial differences in the prevalence of ADHD. There is concern, however, that ADHD in children of racial minorities is often misdiagnosed as behavior problems or not diagnosed at all due to lack of available resources.

Boys are diagnosed with ADHD three to four times more often than girls, the same ratio that is seen in tic disorders, learning disabilities, and comorbid disorders that have a high incidence of ADHD associated with them. There is growing suspicion, however, that the incidence in boys and girls may not be so different. ADHD in girls may be missed for several reasons. In general, girls seem to be less active than boys, perhaps in part due to genetics, so that in a social context with boys at play, a girl with ADHD may not stand out as particularly hyperactive, impulsive, or physically aggressive. Also, ADHD can occur without hyperactivity, which may account for the different reported prevalence in boys and girls. Instead of exhibiting hyperactive and impulsive behavior, the child with ADHD-I tends to sit quietly and miss what is going on, and this type of ADHD is diagnosed more often in girls.

Causes of ADHD

The original explanation for ADHD was brain damage that had occurred prior to birth. Physicians coined the terms *minimal brain dysfunction* or *minimal brain damage*, which covered a diverse group of children including those with learning disabilities, low intelligence, and severe behavior problems. Even now that ADHD has been differentiated from learning disabilities and behavior problems, its cause has not been clearly identified. ADHD is a variable disorder with several possible causes, both genetic and environmental.

Genetic Causes

Human cells contain about 25,000 genes, which are made up of the material deoxyribonucleic acid (DNA). DNA is composed of four base compounds (adenine, thymine, cytosine, and guanine), and the sequences of these bases supply the genetic codes for all the body's proteins. Variations in these sequences are associated with differences in physical appearance, personality, behavior, intelligence, and disease vulnerability. Alterations in the bases, such as the substitution of one for another or the addition of deletion of one or more, are called *mutations*. Scientists have discovered that ADHD is associated with certain gene mutations.

In all human cells except eggs and sperm, genes are present in two copies, one from each parent. Dominant genetic disorders occur when a mutation in only one copy of a gene is sufficient to cause the disorder, whereas a recessive genetic disorder requires two mutant copies of the gene for the disorder to arise. *Penetrance* is a term for the percentage of individuals who inherit a mutated gene and manifest the resulting disease. In dominant genetic disorders, if everyone who inherits at least one copy of the mutated gene has the disease, then there is 100 percent penetrance; incomplete penetrance occurs when not all of the people who inherit a copy of the mutated gene develop the disease. In recessive genetic disorders, incomplete penetrance occurs when not all of the people who inherit both copies of the mutated gene develop the disease.

Although a genetic predisposition for ADHD has been demonstrated through family, adoption, and twin studies, the child of a parent with ADHD will not necessarily develop the disorder. There is also great variability in the symptoms present and their severity, which suggests that mutations in several genes may be at work in ADHD.

A common thread of learning or behavioral problems often exists in the family of someone diagnosed with ADHD. Careful inspection of the family history typically reveals a close relative with ADHD or ADHD-like symptoms. When compared to the general population, an estimated four- to eight-fold increased risk for ADHD exists among the immediate family members of an individual with ADHD.

The most compelling evidence of a genetic cause for ADHD comes from twin studies. When studying the family histories of children with behavioral disorders, there is not always a clear inheritance pattern. Many conditions are the result of the interaction of genetic mutations and environmental factors. Twin studies, which can control for prenatal environmental influences, are used to determine the impact of genes on human behavior. Both identical and fraternal twins share similar prenatal and in most cases postnatal environments, but only identical twins share the same genes, whereas fraternal twins have about 50 percent of their genes in common, the same as other full-siblings. Thus, by comparing the concordance rates (the likelihood that one twin will have the disorder if the other twin is affected) of identical and fraternal twins, researchers can estimate the genetic contribution to the condition being studied. Wendy Sharp and colleagues at the National Institute of Mental Health found a 90 percent concordance rate for ADHD in identical twins. In the remaining 10 percent of twins who were not both affected, there was a greater likelihood of breech presentation, low birth weight (one twin may have received fewer nutrients in utero), and other "unspecified environmental influences."

Research is ongoing to identify the genes responsible for ADHD. One of the major candidates is the D4 dopamine receptor gene, which is located on chromosome 11. The D4 receptor binds to the neurotransmitters dopamine, epinephrine, and norepinephrine, so that a person with a mutation in this gene would have abnormal nerve signals in the brain. A mutation on chromosome 16 has also been linked to ADHD. According to a study by Dr. Susan Smalley, siblings with ADHD have a strong chance of sharing this mutation. Mutations in the same region of chromosome 16 also have been implicated in autism, leading to speculation that changes in this chromosome region may contribute to the common deficits of inattention and hyperactivity found in both ADHD and autism.

Based on these studies, it appears likely that mutations in several genes cause a predisposition for ADHD. The exact symptoms and their severity are variable, however, due to the effects of incomplete penetrance as well as prenatal and postnatal environmental factors. A diagnosis of ADHD should never be made based on genetic testing alone. Although an individual may have a mutation in one of these "ADHD genes," if symptoms do not exist, then the disorder is not present.

Known Environmental Causes

Genetics plays a large part in the development of ADHD, but genes alone do not account for all cases. Environmental causes have also been shown to be factors in some ADHD cases. Smoking and alcohol use during pregnancy and increased blood lead levels either from fetal exposure, ingestion, or inhalation in young children increase the risk of developmental problems, ADHD, and learning difficulties. In addition, injury while in the uterus due to high blood pressure or infection in the mother as well as infection or injury after birth have all been implicated as potential causes of ADHD.

Tobacco. Several studies have confirmed that smoking a half pack of cigarettes or more per day during pregnancy can adversely affect a child's learning and behavior. A study at the Mount Sinai School of Medicine showed that mothers who smoked during pregnancy rated their toddlers as having more negative behaviors including impulsiveness, risk-taking, and rebelliousness than mothers who had not smoked during pregnancy. Decreased scores in reading comprehension and language skills (particularly auditory processing) and increased levels of hyperactivity also have been found in patients whose mothers smoked during pregnancy. A Danish study reported that women who smoked more than a half pack of cigarettes per day during pregnancy had a three-fold risk of having a child with ADHD, and these results could not be explained by differences in parental socioeconomic status, delivery complications, family history, or other behavioral problems. A National Institutes of Health study found the risk to be even greater: children whose mothers smoked during pregnancy had four times the risk of having ADHD than the general population, even when parental ADHD, parental IQ, and socioeconomic status were taken into account.

Alcohol. Consuming as few as two drinks per day during pregnancy may cause adverse affects on the infant, and more severe problems appear as the amount of alcohol intake increases. The timing of the alcohol exposure during the forty weeks of pregnancy also has an effect: if exposure is high in the first part of the pregnancy, physical abnormalities are more likely. Fetal alcohol spectrum disorder (FASD) is the name given to the diverse range of symptoms in children with a history of alcohol exposure during the prenatal period. Each year as many as 40,000 babies are born in the United States with FASD, and ADHD and mood disorders are commonly diagnosed in these children. Affected children are typically irritable as young infants and hyperactive as toddlers. As for the physical effects, FASD children tend to have low birth weight and small head size without catch-up growth, thus the children tend to remain small for their age.

Lead. Elevated lead levels in the blood are harmful to humans, especially children. Increased lead levels have been linked to a higher risk of ADHD, and high levels are known to cause significant behavior problems, learning disabilities, hearing loss, and at very high levels convulsions, coma, and even death. Toddlers are more vulnerable to the effects of lead poisoning due to their rapidly growing and developing brains. During this important time of brain growth, maturation of nerve connections and organization of nerve pathways occur, and these processes can be disrupted by the toxic effects of lead.

The exact level at which children are adversely affected is not known. The level of concern for young children, pregnant women, and nursing mothers is 10 micrograms of lead per deciliter (usually noted µg/dl) of blood. If an individual shows such a level, an investigation of possible sources of lead should take place and a follow-up assessment of lead level in the blood should be made. Although there is no known safe level of lead in the body, medical treatment (chelation) is usually not warranted unless the level is above 45 micrograms per deciliter.

Increased lead levels are more common in young children due to their oral nature. Many toddlers suck on their fingers or other objects that may contain dust, and dust containing lead is a common source of exposure. Lead dust can come from several sources, such as deteriorating lead-based paint used in homes built prior to 1960, deteriorating vinyl blinds purchased before 1997, contaminated soil around old gas stations, or clothing of a parent who is exposed to lead in the workplace. Other sources of lead include pottery (pots from Mexico, Vietnam, and other countries may contain lead), batteries, cosmetics, lead pipes, lead solder, or old plumbing fixtures containing lead.

Potential Environmental Causes

Delivery complications such as breech presentation, prolonged labor, or the umbilical cord becoming wrapped around the infant's neck during delivery (in some cases causing compromised blood flow to the brain) have been implicated as possible causes of ADHD. Low birth weight, meningitis (an infection or inflammation of the tissue that surrounds the brain and spinal cord), and head injury have also been linked to an increased risk of ADHD in a small percentage of individuals. Other suggested, but unproven, environmental factors associated ADHD include low parental education level, poverty, and parenting styles.

Brain Anatomy

Recent studies have focused on abnormal brain anatomy as a cause of ADHD. Through the use of brain imaging technology, including functional magnetic resonance imaging (fMRI), positron emission tomography (PET), and single photon emission computed tomography (SPECT), certain regions of the brain have been identified as different in those with ADHD.

The fMRI is a special type of MRI that allows visualization of the structure of the brain and can measure the activity of the different areas of the brain in response to certain activities. The advantage of this type of scan is that it does not require an injection of dye into the blood stream to visualize the activity levels, instead measuring the differences in oxygen use in the various areas of the brain. Those regions that are active during the completion of a particular task use more oxygen. Researchers have used the fMRI to compare the brain activity of ADHD individuals with that of people without ADHD.

PET and SPECT scans do not provide the clarity of brain structure that the fMRI does. Instead, multicolored images during the scan show the different areas of the brain that are active. These scans are invasive in that they require an injection of a mildly radioactive substance, usually glucose. Active brain cells use more glucose, thus the more intensely colored areas of the brain are the more active ones.

The frontal lobes of the brain, composed of the prefrontal and frontal cortex, make up about one-third of the brain's surface. This region is where higher intellectual functioning, or "executive functions," occur. This region controls the skills that relate to planning, initiating, problem solving, inhibition of impulsivity, and understanding the behavior of others. The frontal lobes also help control voluntary body movements, speech, and, to some degree, mood. The prefrontal area of the frontal lobes is connected to other areas of the brain that are responsible for the control of the neurotransmitters dopamine, norepinephrine, and serotonin. (Further information on neurotransmitters is discussed below). This prefrontal area of the brain appears to be important in the regulation of mood and emotional responses to others. fMRI, PET, and SPECT studies all have shown a lower activity level in the frontal lobes of individuals with ADHD.

Individuals with ADHD also have differences in other areas of the brain involved in the circuits that connect complex motor actions and cognition (thinking and reasoning). Areas that have been implicated include the corpus callosum, the connection between the right and left frontal lobes, which helps the two lobes communicate with each other; the basal ganglia, the interconnected gray masses deep in the cerebral hemisphere, which serve as the connection between the cerebrum; and the cerebellum, which is the center of motor coordination. Figure 2.1 illustrates the areas in the brain that have been shown to be different in patients with ADHD.

Researchers from the National Institute of Mental Health studied children with ADHD and age- and sex-matched

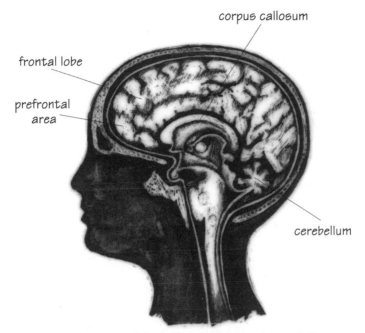

Figure 2.1 Regions of the brain identified as being different in individuals with ADHD.

controls (children without ADHD). The children all underwent brain scans at least twice, some up to four times, over ten years. The ADHD children were found to have smaller volumes by 3 to 4 percent in all of the brain regions mentioned above. This study also showed that ADHD children who were on medication had the same volume of white matter as did the control group, whereas children with ADHD who had never been medicated for the disorder had an abnormally small volume of white matter. The white matter, which thickens as the brain matures, is important in establishing connections between distant brain regions.

Long-term studies using PET scans have shown that differences in the frontal lobes and basal ganglia in individuals with

ADHD disappear following treatment with traditional stimulant medications. Though promising, much research remains to be done before brain imaging can be used to make a diagnosis of ADHD. Safety of the imaging technology and cost effectiveness are also two major concerns that will need to be addressed.

Electroencephalogram Changes. The brain normally produces low-voltage electrical activity that can be measured by the electroencephalogram (EEG). Because there are characteristic EEG recordings at different ages and states of consciousness, it is possible to recognize generalized malfunction of the brain through the use of an EEG. Research on ADHD has also used the quantitative electroencephalogram (qEEG), which performs a computerized evaluation of the level of brain wave activity in different areas of the brain hemispheres. Recent qEEG studies of Australian children and adolescents with ADHD found evidence of increased theta and decreased alpha and beta waves. An increase in theta waves is associated with extreme drowsiness and onset of sleep. Alpha waves are generally associated with alertness and normal level of consciousness. Beta waves become more prominent in the frontal area as drowsiness occurs. Thus, children with ADHD have a lower level of alertness due to the increase in theta waves, which are associated with extreme drowsiness. The differences appear to be particularly prominent in the frontal and temporal areas of the brain.

Neurochemicals. Compared to those without the disorder, individuals with ADHD also show differences in brain chemicals. Studies have shown that people with ADHD have lower levels of the neurotransmitters norepinephrine and dopamine, two chemicals in the brain that transmit information across nerve endings. These substances transmit signals from one neuron to the next when they are released into the small space between nerve cells, known as the *synapse.* Thus, the end of the nerve cell releases the neurotransmitter into the synapse, which is then sent to the receiver end of the next nerve cell. The result of this transmission is the movement of signals through the nervous system. Inadequate levels of norepinephrine and dopamine in brain synapses have been implicated as a cause of ADHD symptoms.

Medications that stimulate the central nervous system (discussed in chapter 4) are those most frequently used to treat ADHD. These medications affect the levels of norepinephrine and dopamine, thus strengthening the case for a neurochemical basis of ADHD. Even more convincing evidence comes from studies that have demonstrated changes in brain activity in the prefrontal cortex and other brain areas in individuals with ADHD when treated with central nervous system stimulants.

Unproven Causes for ADHD

Over the years, researchers and physicians have proposed that diet, vitamin deficiency, allergic reactions to certain food additives and preservatives, and even watching too much television may be related to the symptoms of ADHD. Thus far, there is little scientific evidence to show that these are true factors underlying the disorder.

Diet. During the first few years of life, proper nutrition is especially important to support brain development and growth. Fortunately, most children in the United States do not have a significant nutritional deficiency. Undernourished children, however, have difficulties with focusing and paying attention, thus showing some of the symptoms of ADHD. In the mid-1980s, many children with ADHD symptoms were treated with megavitamin therapy, in which they were given nutritional supplements containing at least ten times the recommended daily allowance of vitamins, minerals, and other elements. Some of these children were found to have sustained liver damage, indicating the possible toxic effects of the high-dose vitamin therapy. Due to the concerns of possible harm, the American Academy of Pediatrics Committee on Nutrition issued a formal statement emphasizing that there is no convincing evidence that poor diet is a cause of ADHD and that megavitamin therapy may be harmful.

Food Additives and Preservatives. In the 1970s, the pediatric allergist Benjamin Feingold proposed that certain food additives, including some preservatives, artificial flavors and colors, and salicylates (contained in many fruits and some vegetables), caused hyperactivity and learning disabilities in children. Children with ADHD were placed on an elimination diet, in which one suspected item at a time was removed from the diet to investigate its effect on the symptoms of ADHD. Subsequent studies showed that only 10 percent of children with ADHD demonstrated true allergies to food dyes, and only 2 percent of those placed on the Feingold diet showed consistent behavioral improvement. Allergens may exacerbate the symptoms of ADHD by affecting mood and behavior, but alone they do not cause the disorder. Furthermore, elimination of the allergen is not an effective treatment for ADHD.

Sugar. The findings of one early study suggested that high sugar consumption was linked to hyperactivity, but this study did not take into account the differences in parenting styles, other behavioral problems, or learning disabilities. In spite of these issues, many parents and physicians attempted to treat children with ADHD by complete elimination of refined sugar. Subsequent, more rigorous studies did not confirm that sugar had adverse effects on the symptom of hyperactivity. One well-controlled study did show that in 2 percent of

ADHD children hyperactivity increased slightly when the child was given a high-sugar diet, but the study has not been duplicated. Although there is no evidence that completely eliminating refined sugar is helpful in most ADHD children, there is little doubt that a balanced diet that is low in sugar is the healthiest option, which should be promoted for all children regardless of whether they suffer from ADHD.

Too Much Television. A study of more than 2600 children revealed that the more television very young children watched, the more likely they were at seven years of age to have attentional problems. Although these findings do not directly link watching too much television with ADHD, parents might reduce the risk for attentional problems by limiting their children's television viewing time. The possibility remains that if a child is watching television many hours each day, a skills deficit may develop due to the fact that the child is not required to sustain attention for long periods of time. Rapidly changing scenes in the television programming available to children do not require sustained attention.

Summary

ADHD is the most commonly diagnosed behavioral disorder in childhood. Family history, twin, adoption, and genetics studies show that in most cases there is a substantial genetic component. Environmental issues such as exposure to toxins, meningitis, low birth weight, delivery complications, and brain injury may play a part in the development of ADHD in a small percentage of individuals. Numerous imaging studies have shown that ADHD is associated with brain anatomy and neurochemical abnormalities, pointing to the physical causes underlying the symptoms of this disorder.

3. Making the Diagnosis

"Until I was put on medicine, it was like my brain was trying to listen to a lot of different channels on the radio at once, and I could only hear parts of each one."
—Jeremy, an eleven-year-old with ADHD,
at a follow-up visit

There are no physical findings, laboratory tests, x-rays, or even psychological tests that alone can be used to make the diagnosis of ADHD. Instead, ADHD is usually diagnosed through excluding other possibilities. For the diagnosis to be made correctly, the health-care provider who is completing the evaluation should obtain information from a variety of sources. Parents should ensure that a good strategic plan of evaluation is completed by a provider who is experienced in working with children and adults with this disorder.

Although the DSM-IV criteria aid in making the diagnosis of ADHD, much more is required to attain good diagnostic accuracy. Many other disorders may be the cause of the inattentive or hyperactive behaviors or may coexist with ADHD. To eliminate disorders that can mimic ADHD, such as hearing or vision problems, health problems, sleep disorders, family issues, or other behavioral disorders, an extensive medical history, psychosocial evaluation, and physical and neurological exam must be part of the evaluation process. A psychological and/or speech and language evaluation may also be necessary to determine whether there are problems with intelligence, specific learning disabilities, or language processing.

Concerns about ADHD typically stem from parents, teachers, and childcare providers due to disruptive behaviors, problems with social relationships, academic struggles, and/or poor self-esteem. Once such problems are identified, parents should consult their physician and schedule a parent-teacher meeting to discuss the difficulties and to see if further evaluation is needed. An evaluation for ADHD should be initiated when problem behaviors are significantly impacting the child's performance and well-being. The best way to evaluate a child for ADHD is through a team approach. The team should be composed of the child or teen, parents or primary caretaker, teachers, and physician. A psychologist, social worker, and speech and/or occupational therapist may also be needed, depending on the symptoms present.

The Medical Evaluation

In an attempt to create a uniform process in the evaluation of ADHD, the American Academy of Pediatrics developed a clinical practice guideline. The following five recommendations were published in the May 2000 issue of *Pediatrics*:

> In a six- to twelve-year-old child who presents with inattention, hyperactivity, impulsivity, academic underachievement, or behavior problems, primary care clinicians should initiate an evaluation for ADHD.
> The diagnosis of ADHD requires that a child meet the DSM-IV criteria.
> The assessment of ADHD requires evidence directly obtained from parents or caregivers regarding the core symptoms of ADHD in various settings, the age of onset, durations of symptoms, and degree of functional impairment.
> The assessment of ADHD requires evidence directly obtained from the classroom teacher (or other school professional)

regarding the core symptoms of ADHD, the duration of symptoms, the degree of functional impairment, and coexisting conditions. A physician should review any reports from a school-based multidisciplinary evaluation where they exist, which will include assessments from the teacher or other school-bases professional.

Evaluation of the child with ADHD should include assessment for coexisting conditions.

Following these guidelines alone is not adequate to make the diagnosis of ADHD. Taking the medical history is the most important piece of the evaluation in order to eliminate disorders that mimic or coexist with ADHD. Past illnesses such as ear infections, asthma, allergies, sleep disorders, and other common problems can also interfere with the child's general well-being and academic functioning. Medications should be reviewed, as some may cause inattention or hyperactivity.

Questions about behavior, school function, social and family adjustment, and social interaction should be covered. Valuable clues can be gained from information not only from parents, but also from the child and teachers. Information from parents will supply important facts such as onset, duration, and the severity of symptoms as well as the traditional medical information that is needed. The child or teen can often relate important information that the parents may not know. Exploration of depressive symptoms, drug use, sleep problems, or other mood disorders such as anxiety should be covered with both the parents and the child. Children or teens may not recognize their own behaviors, such as withdrawal from a group of friends, as being a symptom of depression, whereas parents and teachers may better describe what they are seeing in the child.

Many questions should be covered when evaluating the possible reasons for inattention or school problems. The following are some standard questions that a physician may ask parents:

When did you first notice that your child was having problems?
Do problems exist anywhere other than school?
Has your child ever repeated a grade or been in danger of failing?
Does your child receive any special services in school?
Do the problems seem to occur at any particular time of the day or during a particular class?
How are your child's grades?
Have the teachers complained of any behavior problems?
Do you think that your child could really do the work if he were able to sit still?

Questions that a child or teen may be asked include:

Are you having any problems with learning in school?
Do you have problems paying attention in class?
Do you think that you could do the work if you were able to concentrate?
Do you have problems completing your work?
Do you ever feel sad or anxious about school?
Do you have any problems falling asleep?
Do you fall asleep in class?
How are things going socially?
Do you or any of your friends use alcohol or drugs?

These are only a few of the questions that might be asked, and other questions may arise depending on the answers to these questions.

The family history, a review of health and school problems of other family members, is very important in light of the genetic information that is known about ADHD. Because relatives may never have received an actual diagnosis of ADHD, it is important to gather information about symptoms that have occurred in family members, including behavior problems, school difficulties, academic failure, and abnormal moods. Common questions that are asked about family history include:

Did you or your spouse have any problems in school?
Is there anyone in the family with a history of learning disabilities, speech problems, or attentional problems?
Are there any family members with mood problems such as depression, anxiety, anger control issues, or bipolar disorder?
Do any family members have problems with drug or alcohol addiction?

The psychosocial history, or the evaluation of home life, is another important part of the assessment. A recent move, family separation, divorce, death, or other significant events could effect concentration in anyone. A child who is experiencing ongoing violence in the home (either witnessing spousal abuse or experiencing the abuse himself) will likely have problems paying attention in school due to the mental and possibly physical injuries that he is dealing with.

Teacher information is imperative in making the diagnosis of ADHD. Although there are times when a teacher may not note the inattention in a well-behaved child due to classroom size or the behavior of others, if there are no problems noted in school such as incomplete work or missed instructions, the diagnosis of ADHD is unlikely. A review of teacher notes, report cards, standardized tests, and schoolwork can be key in determining the extent and severity of the problems.

Differences among schools, such as classroom size and arrangement, student numbers, teacher knowledge of ADHD, teaching style, and level of academic difficulty, can have an impact on a child's classroom performance. For instance, a child who has moved from a school with a classroom of twelve children to a classroom of twenty-five may have sudden problems with incomplete work and missed instructions. In the smaller classroom, the attentional problems may have been present, but less noticeable. A lower teacher-to-student ratio is helpful to the ADHD child due to the likelihood of more individualized instruction. Another reason for increased problems with inattention and hyperactivity may be a move to a school that is more difficult academically or to one with a different level of understanding of ADHD. Open classrooms, those in which there are several teaching centers in one large room, can be a very difficult surrounding for a child with inattention because of the many distractions that cannot be filtered out.

Vision and hearing screenings should be completed on all individuals suspected of having ADHD. A child's development, learning, attention span, and general social interaction can be markedly influenced by vision or hearing impairment. The earlier the onset of the problem, the greater the impact will be on the child. Young children may not know that their vision or hearing is different than others, because there is no reference point of what is normal. Children referred for problems with school performance or inattention are regularly found to have a mild hearing or vision deficit.

Once the history is complete, a physical examination is performed on the child to look for signs of physical or neurological abnormalities that might contribute to the behavior or learning problems. A tremor or shakiness may alert the doctor to a possible thyroid problem. A child with fluid behind his eardrum may need a formal hearing test. Large tonsils and noisy breathing noted during the exam may indicate the need for further evaluation by an ear, nose, and throat specialist.

Laboratory Tests

There are no routine laboratory tests that are specifically recommended in the evaluation of ADHD. Blood tests may be ordered if the medical history or physical examination suggests an underlying medical condition. If the child has a poor diet or a poor appetite, then a complete blood count may be ordered to check for anemia, a deficiency in number and/or abnormal size of red blood cells. Iron-deficiency anemia, often due to poor nutrition in children, has been linked to problems with development and learning.

A family history of thyroid problems and a tremor noted in the child would likely initiate a thyroid function test. An overactive thyroid may cause jitteriness or shakiness, sleep problems, and irritability, whereas an underactive thyroid may cause increased drowsiness, problems with constipation, and slowness in movement, thinking, and processing information.

Staring spells, which may be a sign of a seizure disorder, may dictate the need for an EEG. Abnormal findings on the neurological exam such as significant motor abnormalities could cause the examiner to order an MRI or CT scan.

The Psychological Evaluation

Grade repeats, academic struggles, or poor performance on group standardized tests dictate the need for psychological testing. Intelligence and academic testing completed with the child, one-on-one, will be helpful in determining whether a learning disability or a low IQ is the cause of the problems. Children with ADHD often score poorly in group testing situations because they are not paying attention, working quickly, and staying on task; therefore, they either miss instructions or do not complete the test. The rules of group standardized tests do not allow the teacher to prompt the student to get back to work or to repeat instructions to ensure that the student understands them.

Tests of intelligence (psychometric tests) attempt to measure the factors that make up intelligence. The original test of intelligence was developed to identify children who were unable to handle academic work and who should be removed from regular classes and given more help. Today the tests are also used to discover unusually gifted children who may need enrichment in their programming. Psychometric tests are used to assess the level of cognitive abilities (thinking and reasoning), and the Stanford-Binet Intelligence Scale and Wechsler Intelligence Scale are two intelligence tests that are commonly used when evaluating a person's innate intelligence. The tests are divided into two major areas of intelligence, verbal skills and performance or puzzle-solving skills. A child's performance is evaluated on the basis of age, because as a child grows older their abilities increase as well. The scores are compared with standardized norms or normative values, scores that have been determined to be normal for a child at a particular age based on a large sample of children. Intelligence tests are sometimes necessary to understand the appropriate expectations that should be placed on the child.

Tests of academic achievement are designed to measure the level of a child's academic skills. Areas that are tested include: sight word reading, reading comprehension, spelling, written and oral expression (the ability to put thoughts into words), listening comprehension, and mathematical skills such as the ability to identify and write numbers, solve basic mathematical operations, and solve word problems. A lack of exposure to material can significantly affect scores on these academic tests. For example, a five-year-old child who has never had anyone read to him or work with him on letters, numbers, or colors will start school behind his more experienced peers. A child who has missed several months of school due to illness would be at a disadvantage in academic achievement testing simply due to the missed instructional time. Some of the tests that are used include the Wide Range Achievement Test, Wechsler Individual Achievement Test, and the Kaufman Achievement Test. The scores from these tests also have standardized normative values to which they can be compared.

As part of the psychological evaluation, the clinician will typically use rating scales completed by both teachers and parents, and in cases of teens and adults, self-rating scales are often obtained (Table 3.1). These scales attempt to separate out the symptoms of inattention and hyperactivity from oppositional behavior, poor social skills, and aggression. The Child Behavior Checklist and other similar scales were devised to evaluate the child's or teen's overall functioning. This scale separates internalizing symptoms such as anxiety, depression, or obsessive feelings from those externalizing behaviors such as hyperactivity, impulsivity, and aggression.

Continuous performance tests are very simple tasks that require the individual being evaluated to look at a computer screen and watch for a certain pattern to occur. The instruction may be as simple as "Each time you see the letter X followed by the letter O, hit the space bar." The tasks are designed to measure the amount of inattention, impulsivity, and vigilance exhibited during a particular time frame. The test results yield the number of correct hits (attention to task),

Table 3.1 Rating Scales Used in the Evaluation of ADHD

Scale	Key Areas Evaluated	Teacher Form	Parent Form	Self-rating Form
Conners-Revised (CRS-R)	inattention, hyperactivity, oppositional behavior, anxiety, perfectionism, social problems	yes	yes	yes, for ages 12–17
ADD-H: Comprehensive teacher rating scale and parent form (ACTeRS)	inattention, hyperactivity, social skills, oppositional behavior	yes	yes	
Swanson, Nolan, and Pelham Checklist (SNAP)	inattention, hyperactivity, oppositional, aggressive, and impulsive behaviors, social problems	yes	yes	
NICHQ Vanderbilt Assessment Scale	inattention, hyperactivity, oppositional and conduct problems, anxiety, depression	yes	yes	
Attention Deficit Disorders Evaluation Scale, 3rd edition (ADDES-3)	inattention, hyperactivity, impulsivity	yes	yes	
Child Behavior Checklist	depression, anxiety, obsessive compulsive behaviors, tic disorders, inattention, aggression, conduct problems, hyperactivity (not as sensitive for ADHD, but a good tool to evaluate other symptoms)	yes	yes	yes, for ages 12–17

the number of incorrect hits (impulsively hitting when the pattern is not there), and the number of times the pattern was missed (vigilance or ability to stay on task). Although continuous performance tests alone are not a good screening tool for ADHD, they are sometimes used in addition to rating scales and other testing.

An evaluation by a speech pathologist may be necessary if there are concerns about the verbal skills of the individual. Language skills can then be compared with the IQ score to determine whether specific language problems exist. There are two major areas of language development: expressive language, the ability to express one's thoughts in understandable language, and receptive language, the ability to understand and interpret what is being said. An auditory processing disorder, which is a receptive language problem, is often confused with ADHD. In this disorder the child can hear the words but is unable to interpret them correctly; thus, the child will seem to be either hearing impaired or inattentive.

Disorders that Mimic ADHD

A child's success in school depends on his academic abilities, emotional well-being, social interaction, classroom behavior, school attendance, and physical health. Most disorders that mimic ADHD cause difficulty with attention span, but some disorders can also cause hyperactivity and/or impulsivity. Delay of proper identification and treatment of ADHD look-alikes could be detrimental to the individual and may cause significant long-term consequences.

ADHD look-alikes include medical disorders, mental disorders, learning disorders, psychosocial problems, and behavioral disorders. Anyone of these disorders can cause many of the symptoms of ADHD. It is also important to keep in mind that each of these problems discussed below can coexist with ADHD and, if left undiscovered, can make the ADHD more difficult to treat.

Medical Disorders

Sleep Disorders. Twenty to 30 percent of children have sleep-related problems that are significant enough to impact the family. Over one-third of children with sleep problems have increased behavioral and emotional symptoms when compared to those without sleep problems. Children who do not get adequate sleep at night often have difficulty paying attention in class, and fidgety and impulsive behaviors are common symptoms. Snoring, nightmares, night terrors, waking in the middle of the night, bed-wetting, and problems with sleep settling can all be culprits in decreasing a child's restful sleep.

Another problem common to teens is that if they are left to their own natural sleep/wake cycle, the cycle will shift forward. Compared to younger children, teens will sleep later in the morning and stay up later at night. Thus, teens tend to have difficulty falling asleep early enough to allow for an adequate night of sleep, as most teens need at least eight hours of sleep each night. To help combat this issue, some high schools have changed the start time for students to later in the morning and dismiss the students later in the day. A later dismissal will usually decrease the amount of time that teens are left unsupervised, thus solving two common problems with one change.

Sleep settling problems often coexist with ADHD, thus the sleep history should be addressed for every child suspected of having this disorder. Consuming drinks with caffeine, such as soft drinks, coffee, or tea, in the evening may interfere with sleep settling. Children who do not have a good bedtime routine (discussed further in chapter 5) may need to have a regular bedtime established. Children should not be allowed to fall asleep in front of a television because it is too stimulating and will often delay sleep. Video games are even worse offenders. The solutions to the sleep problems may be simple, but in some cases such as severe snoring, a visit to an ear, nose, and throat specialist or to a sleep lab may be necessary to rule out sleep apnea, a repetitive, several-second pause in breathing during sleep.

Chronic Illnesses. Almost half of those children with chronic illnesses will have school-related problems, including an inability to concentrate and mood changes. Common illnesses that can cause frequent school absences include migraine headaches, asthma, and allergies. Numerous school absences can cause further problems with school performance and academic achievement. The missed classroom instruction and assignments may lead to additional difficulties and frustration upon the return to school.

The treatment of the illness can also affect a child's ability to perform well in school. Medications can interfere with attention and concentration or even cause hyperactivity, including some seizure, asthma, or allergy medications (Table 3.2). The medications that the individual is taking and the potential side effects must be reviewed in individuals with symptoms of ADHD. The culprit may be medicine and not true ADHD.

Seizure Disorders. Partial or absence seizures may be difficult to recognize. These seizures typically last a few seconds to a couple of minutes and may include a brief episode of eye-blinking, lip-smacking, or staring and posturing. A child with a seizure disorder may sit and stare for brief periods

Table 3.2 Common Medications that May Cause Symptoms of ADHD

	Trade Name	Side Effects that Mimic ADHD
Allergy Medications		
Pseudoephedrine HCl	numerous cold and allergy medications	problems falling asleep, nervousness, agitation
Asthma Medications		
Albuterol	Ventolin, VoSpire, AccuNeb	nervousness, shakiness, restlessness, problems falling asleep
Theophylline	Theodur, Uniphyl, Unicontin	nervousness, problems falling asleep, anxiety
Seizure Medications		
Oxcarbazepine	Trileptal	sleepiness, feelings of tiredness, confusion, speech or language problems, problems with concentration
Phenobarbital	Luminal	sleepiness, hyperactivity, problems with concentration
Phenytoin	Dilantin	nervousness, mental confusion, problems falling asleep
Topiramate	Topamax	difficulty with memory, problems talking, feelings of tiredness, nervousness, difficulty with concentration, anxiety
Valproic acid	Depakene, Depakote	sleepiness, problems falling asleep, shakiness, problems thinking

and then appear confused or "out of it" if touched by someone. During these often-unnoticed episodes, the child may
miss instruction and seem to lose his place, which are symptoms shared by children with ADHD-I.

Mental Disorders

Several mental disorders can be difficult to differentiate
from ADHD. In this section, I describe those most common
in children and explain the similarities and differences
between these mental disorders and ADHD.

Depression. Depression is defined as an individual exhibiting a depressed mood most of the day every day for a period
of at least two weeks. Any individual who is depressed has a
diminished ability to concentrate. In children and adolescents
suffering from depression, the mood may be irritable rather
than depressed. Sleep problems such as inability to fall asleep
or an excessive need for sleep may also be present. A depressed
mood can be compounded by the fatigue from poor sleep and
is often misinterpreted as laziness or lack of motivation. The
restlessness that accompanies depression may appear to be
hyperactivity and the slowness in movement can be inter-
preted as inattention, which may cause suspicion of ADHD
in depressed individuals.

Bipolar or Manic Depressive Disorder. In years past, bipolar
disorder was rarely diagnosed in the young child; however, new
information has revealed that this disorder does exist in children. Bipolar disorder is defined as a combination of manic
and depressive episodes, and the presentation can be easily
confused with ADHD. A manic episode is a distinct period of
abnormally and persistently elevated or expansive or irritable
mood. While in these episodes, the person will be grandiose

with inflated self-esteem. During a manic phase, an adult may accrue huge shopping bills whether money is available or not or may engage in nonstop writing or painting. A child with bipolar disorder may manifest the grandiosity by trying to tell his teachers or coaches how to do their jobs. Compared to hyperactivity of ADHD, a child with mania has an increased involvement in goal-directed activity. There is often agitation both emotionally and in a motor sense, if the goal-directed activity is not accomplished. In a child with ADHD, however, the hyperactivity is not goal directed. Other symptoms of bipolar disorder that can be confused with ADHD include decreased need for sleep or an excessive involvement in pleasurable activities with a high potential for painful consequences.

Anxiety Disorder. Symptoms of anxiety disorder include restlessness, tiredness, trouble concentrating, irritability, muscle tension, and disturbed sleep, and many of these symptoms can mimic those of ADHD. Anxiety disorder is among the most common of childhood psychiatric disorders and may affect up to 15 percent of children and teens. Whiney, irritable behavior and refusal to attend school or difficulty with separation from parents are other clues that there is more to school problems than inattention.

Adjustment Disorder. This is a relatively common disorder that is a constellation of emotional or behavioral problems in response to some type of stressor that the child has experienced. The stressor could be a divorce, a move, the death of a close relative, or a chronic illness in a caretaker. Inattention, poor sleep, or behavioral difficulties can arise in children with adjustment disorder. The results of an adjustment disorder can be significant problems with emotion, conduct, and/or poor academic performance.

Asperger's Syndrome. This syndrome is included in the autism-spectrum disorders. The essential features of Asperger's syndrome include a severe impairment of social interaction that includes poor use of nonverbal behaviors such as body language or facial expressions, poor peer relationships, and a very limited repertoire of behaviors, interests, and activities. Although these children typically have no problems with intelligence, language development, or large motor skills development, their spoken language may seem odd due to the stiffness of speech, lack of voice inflection, and lack of understanding of jokes. Children with Asperger's syndrome are usually judged to be somewhat clumsy, both physically and socially. Because of their poor social interaction and lack of social awareness, these individuals often are viewed as inattentive and function poorly in a traditional classroom setting.

Learning Disorders

A learning disability is diagnosed when a child's academic achievement on individually administered standardized tests is significantly below what would be expected for the child's age, education, and level of intelligence. A learning disability can occur in reading, mathematics, writing, or language skills. Language problems usually present before the other learning disabilities and can put a child at risk for other learning problems.

Early signs of a learning disability may include delayed speech; difficulty following directions; delays in the development of fine motor skills, such as buttoning or tying shoes; and poor memory skills, such as problems with learning the alphabet, trouble differentiating right from left, or a dislike of learning to read or write. These children are often mistaken as having ADHD. In a regular classroom, a child with a learning disability will appear inattentive because the work being covered is beyond his skill level. As the child gets older, he also may appear hyperactive and impulsive, turning into the class clown to divert attention from the fact that he is having trouble learning.

Help for these children can include one-on-one tutorial services and special classes. Because a broad range of learning disabilities exists, each child should be treated as an individual and have the programming set up for his or her personal needs. There is a high rate of depression and school dropout in teens with these disorders, and research has shown a link between ADHD and learning disabilities.

Psychosocial Problems

Another reason for academic difficulties in children is psychosocial problems in the family. Although psychosocial problems can be related to the issues of adjustment disorder, the difference is that it is the situation itself—not the child's adjustment to it—that is affecting the child. For instance, a chaotic home may not afford the opportunity for a child to appropriately prepare for school. Violence in the home can cause more significant school problems. The violence might be directed at the mother by the father or vice versa, or the abuse may be directed at the child or another sibling. A child who lives in a violent home is often preoccupied by these issues and suffers from fear and anxiety while trying to anticipate what is going to happen next. Psychosocial issues such as these can cause any child to have symptoms that mimic the disorganized, forgetful behavior of a child with ADHD.

Different parenting styles may also cause problem behaviors in children, or they may cause some normal behaviors to be perceived as problematic. In their book *Disruptive Behavior Disorder in Children*, psychologists Michael Breen and Thomas Altepeter noted that outside issues can affect parenting styles, such as marital stress, financial problems, and psychiatric illnesses in the parents. Another issue to consider is that some children are easier to parent than others. Some children are naturally more passive or laid-back, whereas others are more active and strong-willed. Although all of these represent normal behaviors in children, they take different parenting approaches. If parents do not have the skills in their armament to appropriately parent their child's particular temperament or behavior, they may attend parenting classes, which can teach good management skills for active, strong-willed children.

Behavioral Disorders

Several behavioral disorders are frequently misidentified as ADHD. Any of these behavior disorders can coexist with ADHD, but they may also occur alone.

Substance Abuse. Children with ADHD are at a threefold higher risk for substance abuse. Thus, a teen with ADHD who has done well with treatment of ADHD and suddenly begins to develop the warning signs of substance abuse should have this possibility investigated. General warning signs of substance abuse include withdrawn behaviors, memory loss, mood swings, a negative change in appearance, explosive behavior, disregard for rules, absenteeism from school, and running away from home. A sudden drop in grades or change in behavior in a teen that has performed well in the past should prompt an investigation of substance abuse.

Many drugs are readily available to teens. Alcohol is the most available and cheapest drug abused by teens. Behavioral changes documented in adolescents with chronic alcohol use include a drop in grades, increased absenteeism, decreased performance in sports, change in friends, and lethargy or mood changes. Acute use of marijuana has been shown to cause impaired memory and inattention. Chronic effects may include a decrease in mathematics skills, verbal expressive abilities, and problems with selective memory retrieval.

Oppositional Defiant Disorder. This disorder is a recurrent pattern of defiant, disobedient, and negative behaviors toward all authority figures, not just to the parents. These behaviors fall outside typical parenting or temperament issues. Specific behaviors that might be confused with ADHD include refusing to comply with the requests of adults, displaying deliberately annoying behaviors, and being touchy and irritable and easily annoyed by others. In a child with ADHD, however, there is not open defiance; the child's behaviors are due to the inattention and impulsivity. Up to 35 percent of children with ADHD will also have oppositional defiant disorder.

Conduct Disorder. The most serious of the behavioral disorders seen in children is conduct disorder. Though typically seen in teens, conduct disorder can occur prior to adolescence. Children with this disorder violate major societal rules and the rights of others, deliberately destroy property, steal, and lie. Early onset of drug use and sexual acting out are also common. These teens frequently have a history of oppositional defiant disorder with inadequate or ineffective intervention given when they were younger. Conduct disorder can coexist with ADHD. If a child or teen shows signs of conduct disorder, placement in behavioral therapy is a must.

Summary

Because a myriad of other medical and behavioral disorders can mimic ADHD, it is important to have a child properly evaluated. The appropriate diagnosis of a child's school or behavioral problems can be made by a careful investigation of all aspects of the child's life. A complete evaluation for ADHD should include a carefully taken history, observation of and interaction with the child, a complete physical and neurological evaluation, and hearing and vision testing. School information should also be obtained, including the behaviors observed by teachers as well as grades and academic achievement test scores. Once gathered, all of this information will help to evaluate whether the child's primary problem is ADHD or some type of medical, mental, psychological, or behavioral disorder or a learning disability.

4. Treatment

"I went home and cried after our first visit. Finally, I had a reason for my son's problems. Now I have hope!"
—Words from a mother about the diagnosis of her son's ADHD

The success rate in the treatment of ADHD is excellent. Up to 80 percent of those with ADHD will have a positive response to medication alone. No single treatment is right for everyone, however, and the variability of academic skills, intelligence, school placement, behavioral issues, parenting skills, and coexisting conditions make it important to fashion an individual treatment plan for each person diagnosed with ADHD.

The Treatment Process

In an effort to help guide physicians in the treatment of children and teens with ADHD, in 2001 the American Academy of Pediatrics developed the "Clinical Practice Guideline: Treatment of School-Aged Children with ADHD." The guideline provides general recommendations and emphasizes the need to consider the variable backgrounds and symptoms of those with ADHD. The following recommendations were made in the guidelines:

> Primary care clinicians should establish a management program that recognizes ADHD as a chronic condition.

The treating clinician, parents, and child, in collaboration
with school personnel, should specify appropriate target
outcomes to guide management.

The clinician should recommend stimulant medication
and/or behavioral therapy, as appropriate, to improve
target outcomes in children with ADHD.

The clinician should periodically provide a systematic
follow-up for the child with ADHD. Monitoring should
be directed to target outcomes and adverse effects by
obtaining specific information from parents, teachers,
and the child.

Although medication is the cornerstone of treatment for
most people with ADHD, a multifaceted approach is often
needed to address parental or personal preferences, coexisting
disorders, and environmental issues. Behavior or family problems should be treated with counseling, and specific academic
problems should be addressed with tutoring or classroom
accommodations. Coexisting disorders may require treatment
from other specialists, such as speech or occupational therapists. By fashioning an individualized treatment plan, a better
outcome is more likely.

Empowerment through Knowledge

The demystification and clarification process is the first
step in an appropriate treatment plan for ADHD. Although
ADHD is a well-identified disorder, many parents and children are regularly told that problems stem from poor parenting or laziness and oppositional behavior in the child. When
the diagnosis of ADHD is made, parents may have feelings of
great relief but also guilt for the frustration and anger that

they have felt toward their child. Children and teens with ADHD usually know that they perform differently from others, and a diagnosis of this disorder will allow them to understand why. Social issues, self-esteem problems, and parent relational problems may exist in some teens with long-standing, untreated ADHD. The knowledge of what ADHD is and the fact that it is a treatable disorder can allay unwarranted fears and empower the parents and children to look forward to a positive treatment outcome.

There are local and national ADHD support groups that meet regularly to voice frustrations, talk about experiences, share resources, and invite experts to give lectures. Another valuable asset of support groups is that they allow people with similar problems to feel less alone in the difficulties that they are experiencing. Contact information for some of these support groups is provided in the appendix.

Team Building and Goal Setting

The next step is to organize a treatment team. The central members of the team should be the parents, child, physician, teachers, and, in most cases, a psychologist. Other members of the team may include childcare providers, behavior and education therapists, a speech pathologist, occupational therapist, or social worker, as deemed necessary. Baseline information on the child that includes areas of deficiencies and skills should be available to each member of the team. Although a face-to-face meeting with the teachers may not be possible, teacher information is needed to determine problem areas not only in academics but also in peer relationships while at school. Many teachers will appreciate the opportunity to help improve the behavioral problems of students with ADHD.

Parents should discuss the goals of treatment with their physician, and appropriate therapies should be chosen to achieve these goals depending on the child's impairments and needs. Target outcomes that have been suggested by the American Academy of Pediatrics' guidelines include improved relationships with family, peers, and teachers; decreased disruptive and negative behaviors; improved academic performance; increased independence in homework and self-care; improved self-esteem; and improved attention to personal safety. Teens are more likely to cooperate with the therapy if they understand the goals and are included in the decision-making process.

Implementation of Therapy

Consistency of therapy and medical follow-up is necessary for a successful outcome. There should be frequent monitoring of the child's progress by the primary treating provider, that is, the physician or nurse practitioner, if treated medically, or other provider as appointed by the team. This progress information is obtained through regular parent and teacher rating scales and school records, such as grades and achievement scores. Several of the rating scales listed in Table 3.1 include self-rating scales for teens and adults. When behavioral or other therapies are implemented, input from the providers of those therapies will also help determine the progress being made and the need for continued or additional treatment.

Medication Treatment

Factors that must be considered and discussed between parents and physicians prior to the initiation of medication treatment include the potential benefits versus risks and possible adverse effects, the potential interactions with other prescription and over-the-counter medications, and the anticipated costs incurred with medication use. A frank discussion should occur regarding what the medication can and cannot do. For example, some children have the notion that the medications are "be smart" or "be good" pills, when in fact the medications simply help an ADHD child pay attention so that his natural intelligence and goodness can shine through. A clear understanding of how the medication works to help with attention, concentration, and impulsivity will help dispel the misinformation.

The medications that have been shown to be effective in the management of ADHD can be divided into three major categories: the central nervous system stimulants; nonstimulant medications such as norepinephrine reuptake inhibitors; and drugs that have not been approved by the Food and Drug Administration (FDA) for use in the treatment of ADHD, so-called off-label medications, such as tricyclic antidepressants and antihypertensive agents.

Central Nervous System Stimulant Medication

In 1937 the psychiatrist Charles Bradley discovered that Benzedrine (amphetamine) had a calming affect on hyperactive children. Since that time, several hundred studies have been completed on the use of central nervous system stimulant medications, which include the amphetamines and methylphenidate, in the treatment of ADHD. Seventy-five to 80 percent of individuals with ADHD have shown an improvement of symptoms when treated with this class of medication. The benefits expected from the stimulants include sustained attention span and decreased impulsivity and hyperactivity. Other positive affects often seen with adequate treatment include decreased impulsive aggression and improvement in handwriting, reading comprehension, persistence of effort, performance in sports, peer relationships, and emotional control.

The pharmacological action of stimulants is through their ability to block the transport of the neurotransmitters dopamine and norepinephrine out of the synapse and back into the nerve cell. This blockade causes more dopamine and norepinephrine to be available in the synapses in the prefrontal cortex and other areas of the brain affected in those with ADHD (Fig. 4.1). Thus, with better transmission of the information, there is better attention and concentration. Although similar, the amphetamines and methylphenidate differ somewhat in their mode of action. In addition to blocking the transporter system, the amphetamines also stimulate the release of the neurotransmitters. This fact may account for why amphetamines work better in some ADHD individuals and methylphenidates work better in others.

The most convincing evidence for stimulant medication treatment comes from the Multimodal Treatment Study of Children with ADHD, a study funded by the National Institute of Mental Health. Eighteen nationally recognized experts in ADHD at six university medical centers and hospitals evaluated the treatments of ADHD. The study included 579 children who were randomly assigned to one of four treatment groups.

The first group received medication management only. During the first month of treatment, an optimal dose of medication for each child was determined. Once this dose was established, the children were then seen monthly for a half-hour visit, during which the prescribing physician spoke with

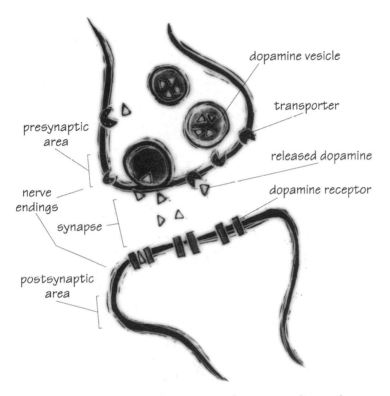

dopamine vesicle

transporter

presynaptic
area

released dopamine

nerve
endings

dopamine receptor

synapse

postsynaptic
area

Figure 4.1 Vesicles carry dopamine to the nerve ending and release it. Transporters then pick up the dopamine and release it into the synapse between two nerve endings. Finally, receptors on the second nerve ending attach to the dopamine, and this nerve passes the neurochemical signal to the next one.

the parent, obtained teacher information, and met with the child to evaluate possible problems with the medication and to give behavioral advice as needed. If the child experienced difficulties that appeared to be related to ADHD medication issues, the physician adjusted the dose.

The second group received behavioral treatment only. Families met up to thirty-five times with a behavior therapist, predominately in group sessions. The therapists made repeated visits to the schools to consult with the children's teachers and to supervise an aide assigned to each child in the group. The children also attended a special eight-week summer treatment program to work on academic, social, and sports skills and to receive intensive behavioral therapy. The therapy lasted up to fourteen months.

The third group received a combination of the medication and behavioral treatments received by groups 1 and 2. The fourth group received routine community care. The children saw the community treatment physician chosen by their parents one to two times per year for short periods of time. The physicians prescribed medication but tended to use low doses of the medication. The community physician did not have contact with the teachers to obtain feedback on how the child was doing.

All the children in this study were evaluated based on classroom performance and teacher and parent rating scales. The study confirmed that ADHD is a medical disorder that can be effectively treated with stimulant medication. The need for close medical follow-up was also verified. The results showed that the medication treatment with close follow-up (group 1) and the combined treatment (group 3) were far superior to the behavioral treatment alone or the routine community care. Although there was not a large difference between the outcomes in groups 1 and 3, in some areas such as anxiety, social skills, academic performance, and parent-child interaction, the combined treatment was slightly superior. The findings were similar across all six research centers, despite the fact that children treated at the different sites had varying sociodemographic characteristics.

In addition to these findings, the Multimodal Treatment Study made several recommendations regarding the treatment of ADHD. Medication effectiveness, appropriate dosing, and the presence of side effects should be evaluated on a regular basis to maximize successful treatment. Frequent follow-ups by the healthcare provider also allow for behavioral or school issues to be discussed as they occur. Conversely, delay in addressing the issues as they occur increases the likelihood of the problem becoming more serious. Finally, frequent visits allow for a better understanding of the disorder and a more effective treatment plan.

There are two primary stimulants that are used in the treatment of ADHD: the amphetamines (Dexedrine, Dextrostat, Adderall, and Adderall XR) and methylphenidate (Ritalin, Ritalin LA, Concerta, Metadate ER, Metadate CD, Focalin, Focalin XR, Methylin, and Daytrana). Table 4.1 lists the duration of action, available dosages, and costs of these stimulant medications. There is no standard dose that is effective for every individual. Some children show improvement at very low doses, whereas others require a much higher dose. All of these medications are classified as schedule II medications by the FDA, which means that they have abuse potential. Although abuse of the medications has not been seen at the low doses used in the treatment of ADHD, physicians and nurse practitioners are charged to carefully monitor the amount of medication dispensed.

These rapid-acting medications can produce a change in behavior within thirty to forty-five minutes after oral ingestion. The short-acting preparations reach maximum effectiveness within two to four hours, and the useful effects wear off within three to six hours. Due to the short duration of action, these medications should be taken at least twice a day to cover the school day, with at least one dose taken at school. The new longer-acting medications, including Concerta, Metadate CD, Ritalin LA, Focalin XR, and Adderall XR, allow the

Table 4.1 Stimulant Medications Used in the Treatment of ADHD

	Duration of action	Available dosages	Cost*	Comments
Amphetamines				
Dextroamphetamine (generic)		5, 10 mg	$	Can be cut in half.
Dexedrine Spansules	6–8 hours	5, 10, 15 mg	$$	
Amphetamine Salts				
Adderall Immediate Release	4 hours	5, 7.5, 10, 12.5, 15, 20, 30 mg	$$$	Can be cut in half
Adderall XR	8–10 hours	5, 10, 15, 20, 25, 30 mg	$$$$	Cannot crush, chew, or half; may sprinkle.**
Methylphenidates				
Methylphenidate (generic)	4 hours	5, 10, 20 mg	$$	
Methylin tablets	4 hours	5, 10, 20 mg	$$	
Methylin liquid	4 hours	5, 10 mg/tsp	$$	
Focalin tablets	4 hours	2.5, 5 mg	$$	
		10 mg	$$$	
Focalin XR	8–10 hours	5, 10, 20 mg	$$$$	Covers the school day; cannot chew or divide, but may sprinkle.**
Metadate ER tablets	6 hours	10, 20 mg	$$	
Ritalin tablets		10, 20 mg	$$	

Ritalin SR	6–8 hours	20 mg	$$	Cannot half, variable duration action.
Metadate CD capsule	8–10 hours	10, 20, 30, 40 mg	$$$	Cannot chew or divide, but may sprinkle.** In each dose, 30 percent immediate release, 70 percent sustained release.
Ritalin LA	8–10 hours	20, 30, 40 mg	$$$	Cannot chew or divide, but may sprinkle.** In each dose, 50 percent immediate release, 50 percent sustained release.
Concerta capsule	8–12 hours	18, 27, 36, 54 mg	$$$$	OROS delivery system, a pump system that allows for a more controlled release of medication. In each dose of the tablet form, 22 percent immediate release. Cannot chew, sprinkle, half, or crush. Should not be used if there is a history of narrowing in the gastrointestinal tract.
Daytrana transdermal patch	11 hours	10, 15, 20, 30 mg	$$$$	Patch is applied each morning and removed 9 hours later. May cause skin irritation or redness.

*Cost per thirty tablets or capsules: $: less than $25; $$: $25–50; $$$: $50–100; $$$$: $100–150

**Sprinkle: If unable to swallow the capsule, OK to open capsule and sprinkle the contents on applesauce; however, chewing the granules will hamper with the delayed absorption of the time-released granules.

individual to be treated with fewer doses that may cover the entire school day and may be helpful in avoiding any stigmatization of the child by other classmates. The FDA recently approved the use of a transdermal patch of methylphenidate (Daytrana), which is effective for eleven to twelve hours, for the treatment of ADHD. At present, it is the only non-oral medication available for the treatment of this disorder.

Common side effects of the central nervous system stimulants include headache, stomachache, decreased appetite with weight loss, and sleep problems. Less common side effects include anxiety, increased agitation, and increased heart rate. This class of medications should not be used in individuals with a diagnosis of psychosis or schizophrenia, glaucoma (increased pressure in the eye), a history of stimulant drug abuse, or a history of cardiac abnormalities such as heart rhythm abnormalities or structural cardiac defects. Concerns have arisen about the cardiac issues due to sudden deaths that have been linked to the use of stimulants, particularly Adderall. In most cases, however, the sudden deaths occurred in individuals with known cardiac disease. Although further research needs to be conducted, a few studies have suggested that stimulants should not be used by individuals with motor tics, because the tics may increase; those with depression, who may have increased problems as the medication wears off; those with anxiety, which may increase with stimulant use; and those with a seizure disorder, unless the seizure disorder is well controlled.

Possible drug interactions with stimulants may include a slower clearance from the body of some blood thinners, such as coumadin, or seizure medications, such as phenobarbital or Dilantin. When the clearance is slower, higher levels of these medications can build up in the body. Therefore, the usual doses may need to be decreased when these medications are used in combination with stimulants. Medicines used for depression, such as tricyclic antidepressants (Elavil, Tofranil, Norpramin) and selective serotonin reuptake inhibitors (Prozac, Paxil, Zoloft, Celexa, Luvox, Lexapro), may also have their clearance affected. Stimulants should not be used with cough and cold medications containing pseudoephedrine (Sudafed and others) due to the risk of an increase in blood pressure and heart rate.

Nonstimulant Medications

Although stimulants are very effective in the treatment of ADHD, these medications do not work for everyone and in some cases should not be used due to other disorders or health problems (see Table 4.1). Nonstimulant medications have been used to treat those who cannot take a stimulant due to side effects, other health issues, or a lack of response to the medication (Table 4.2).

The norepinephrine reuptake inhibitor atomoxetine (Strattera) is the only nonstimulant medication approved by the FDA for the treatment of ADHD. This medication differs from the stimulants in that it is highly specific in inhibiting the reuptake of the neurotransmitter norepinephrine in the synapse. Atomoxetine is not classified as a schedule II drug, which is an advantage in some cases because a new prescription must be written each month for schedule II drugs, whereas refills can be dispensed on an atomoxetine prescription. Unlike the stimulant medications, it typically takes about three weeks of taking atomoxetine to see the full therapeutic effect of the drug. Thus, medication changes should not be made more often than three to four weeks apart.

All the studies that have investigated atomoxetine have shown this medication to be effective in the treatment of ADHD,

Table 4.2   Nonstimulant Medications Used in the Treatment of ADHD

	Duration of action	Available dosages	Cost*	Comments
Selective Norepinephrine Reuptake Inhibitor				
Strattera capsules (atomoxetine)	24 hours	10, 18, 25 mg 40, 60, 80 mg	$$$ $$$$	The only drug listed here that the FDA has approved for treatment of ADHD; takes about three weeks to see the full effect.
Tricyclic Antidepressants				
Tofranil (imipramine)	12 hours	10, 25, 50, 75, 100 mg	$	Not indicated if glaucoma is present; side effects include sleepiness, constipation, dry mouth, an irregular heart rate; very dangerous in overdose.
Centrally Acting Alpha-2 Agonist				
Catapres (clonidine)	8–12 hours	0.1 mg 0.2 mg	$ $$	Abrupt stopping of medication can cause side effects such as a jump in blood pressure or heart rate.

Tenex (guanfacine)	8–12 hours	1, 2 mg	$$	Abrupt stopping of medication can cause side effects such as a jump in blood pressure or heart rate.
Aminoketone Class Antidepressant				
Wellbutrin SR (bupropion)	12 hours	100, 150 mg 200 mg	$$$ $$$$	Same drug that has been used for smoking cessation; not indicated if an eating disorder or seizure disorder is present.
Wellbutrin XL (bupropion)	24 hours	150, 300 mg	$$$$	Same drug that has been used for smoking cessation; not indicated if an eating disorder or seizure disorder is present.

*Cost per thirty tablets or capsules: $: less than $25; $$: $25–50; $$$: $50–100; $$$$: $100–150 although effectiveness comparable to that of stimulants has not been proven. This medication should not be taken by those with coexisting tic disorders, anxiety, or sleep problems. Side effects of atomoxetine include decreased appetite, weight loss, and sleepiness. Among the 2 million people treated with atomoxetine, there have been two reports of toxic effects on the liver, and both individuals recovered when the medication was discontinued. At this time, laboratory monitoring of liver function while on atomoxetine is not deemed necessary.

Off-Label Medications

Many medications that have been used in the treatment of ADHD have not been approved by the FDA for use in children. When a medication has not been approved for use in a particular age group or for a particular disorder, it is called an "off-label" use. Research has shown some positive treatment effects in children for all of the medications described below, although none have been shown to be as effective as the central nervous system stimulants.

In the late 1980s, clonidine (Catapres), a medication commonly used to treat high blood pressure, was found to be beneficial in the management of ADHD. This medication appears to be especially helpful in alleviating the symptoms of impulsivity and hyperactivity. Guanfacine (Tenex), a similarly acting medication, was later found to have similar effects. The mode of action of both clonidine and guanfacine is the inhibition of the release of norepinephrine and increased dopamine reuptake. The changes in behavior may be related to the sedation that the medications produce, although there has been some evidence that guanfacine also improves inattention. In most individuals, neither clonidine nor guanfacine are as helpful as the central nervous system stimulants in the management of ADHD, but they may be effective in those patients who do not respond to the stimulant medications or cannot tolerate their side effects.

Guanfacine has been shown to be more specific in its action on certain brain receptors in the prefrontal cortex. Research has shown that guanfacine improves working memory, reduces distractibility and impulsivity, and improves frustration tolerance. A guanfacine patch has been developed for use in the treatment of ADHD, although it has not yet been approved by the FDA.

Clonidine and guanfacine may be useful in the management of the extreme impulsive anger issues, hyperactivity, and problems with falling asleep. Another group of individuals who may benefit from their use are those who have both ADHD and tic disorders, as these medications are effective in the treatment of tic disorders in some individuals. Side effects include sleepiness, lowering of blood pressure, dizziness, and rarely sleep settling problems. These medications can be dangerous in overdose and should never be abruptly discontinued due to the possibility of a rebound jump in blood pressure. Clonidine causes more problems with sedation and sleepiness, and thus guanfacine may be a better choice in the treatment for those with ADHD.

Modafinil (Provigil) is a stimulant that has FDA approval for the treatment of narcolepsy, a disorder of arousal that causes an awake person to suddenly fall asleep. Studies in both adults and children with ADHD have shown improved short-term and visual memory, spatial planning, vigilance, and task accuracy, and one study reported an overall positive effect in most of the ADHD children treated with modafinil. The manufacturer of Provigil has applied to the FDA for approval of it use for the treatment of ADHD in adults. Side effects may include headaches, nausea, sleep problems, nervousness, anxiety, or dizziness.

Bupropion (Wellbutrin) is a medication that has been used for depression, bipolar disorder, smoking cessation, and ADHD. The mode of action is not yet clear, but it appears to increase the levels of norepinephrine, dopamine, and serotonin levels in the synapses. Although the beneficial effects are not as substantial as those of the central nervous system stimulant medications, several studies have shown that bupropion improves the symptoms of ADHD. Side effects include rashes, nausea, appetite suppression, and sleep problems. In rare cases, seizures have occurred at higher doses, so this medication is not recommended for individuals with a seizure disorder.

The tricyclic antidepressants imipramine (Tofranil) and desipramine (Norpramin) have been used for the management of ADHD symptoms. There is some evidence that tricyclic antidepressants may increase vigilance and decrease impulsivity, and the medications may be helpful in children with coexisting mood, anxiety, or depressive problems. There is no clear evidence that the tricyclic antidepressants are helpful in long-term management of ADHD, however, as the treatment effects appear to diminish over time. Common side effects include drowsiness, dry mouth, and constipation. Cardiac effects that are less common, but tricyclic antidepressants may cause irregular heart beat or rapid heart rate, and these medications can be lethal in overdose due to the cardiac effects.

Counseling

Parental Counseling. Parenting children with ADHD can often be a challenge, especially with a hyperactive and impulsive child. The type of parenting that was successful with other children in the family often does not work for the child with ADHD. Counseling can help parents develop a behavioral management style that is more successful. A cardinal rule in behavior management is "Say what you mean, and mean what you say." A question like "Are you ready to go to bed?" is likely to initiate a negative response, whereas the statement "In fifteen minutes it will be time to take your bath and get ready for bed" is more directive and sets a tone of control. Instructions that may seem to be clear and simple in fact may be too broad for a child with ADHD to successfully complete. For instance, "clean your room" may require more organization and attention skills than some ADHD children possess. The appendix lists some workbooks for parents that cover behavioral management points such as these. When negative parenting patterns are firmly set, however, professional counseling is often necessary.

Behavioral Therapy. Enrollment of children in behavioral therapy may be necessary to help alleviate problems stemming from the ADHD, coexisting disorders, or the reactions of others toward them. Problems with self-esteem, anxiety, oppositional behavior, and social interaction are a few of the issues that can occur in children with ADHD. A trained therapist can help a child learn how to exhibit more appropriate behaviors, develop creative ways to address their problems, and develop respectful behaviors for others.

Play Therapy. For young children with ADHD, play therapy is often used. Play therapy differs from regular play in that a trained therapist helps the child address and resolve problem behaviors or feelings, such as taking turns, following instructions, dealing with frustration, and controlling anger. While involved in a fun activity, it is easier for children to confront and deal with issues that may be bothering them. Compared to talking therapy, play therapy works far better in children under ten years of age. Young children often have no idea of why they act as they do and simply need practice on how to deal with things correctly. If there are other issues such as sadness or anxiety that are affecting the child's behavior, however, those issues may become apparent through play therapy.

Social Skills Training. Formal therapy with a professional who is well versed in social skills training can help a struggling ADHD child or teen to become more adept at approaching social situations. This therapy is best achieved through group practice with peers. Acting out certain social situations with a critique from the therapist will help a child or teen understand appropriate ways to approach different social situations. Some therapist use videotaping during the therapy to help the child better understand appropriate behaviors. While watching a videotape of the acted out situation, the therapist can review with the child the positive points about the interaction and areas that may require improvement.

Psychotherapy. This type of therapy has been shown to improve social skills, peer relationships, and self-esteem in those with ADHD. Psychotherapy works well for those who are ten years and older, have good language skills, and normal intelligence. Often teens and adults with ADHD have had a very difficult time in dealing with their disorder, and signs of anxiety, depression, or anger may be present. Through talking with the therapist, thoughts and feelings that are interfering with normal daily functioning can be addressed. The individual may develop a better understanding of his or her self-defeating patterns of behavior and learn better ways to handle the feelings and situations.

Education Accommodations

Academic success in children and teens with ADHD can often be enhanced by making some relatively simple accommodations in the classroom. The typical issues that recurrently cause problems for school-age children with ADHD include missed instructions, disruptive behaviors, poor note-taking skills, poor performance on timed tests, and difficulty getting homework assignments written down.

The 504 Plan. The Rehabilitation Act of 1973 provided for the 504 Plan. If a child is in a regular public school setting (that is, not in a special education program), the 504 Plan allows an ADHD child to receive special accommodations that will help in some problem areas. To initiate a 504 Plan, the student is first referred by a teacher, support staff (such as the school counselor, psychologist, speech therapist), parent or legal guardian, physician, or therapist. A meeting is held in which a 504 Plan for the student is developed and a review date is set. Some of the accommodations that can be made for the ADHD child include changing the child's seat assignment to a less distracting location, allowing the child to leave the classroom each day for the administration of medication, and adjusting the student's assignments or testing conditions, for instance, by extending the time allowed or modifying the test questions. Significant academic deficits do not have to be present for the child with ADHD to qualify for this plan. Unfortunately, there are no federal monies allocated to schools to help implement the 504 Plan. The interpretation of the law and the services that are given vary from school to school.

Individual with Disabilities Education Act (IDEA). IDEA provides federal guidelines and funding to states to help guarantee special education services to eligible children. To qualify for these services, a child must have significant academic impairments. Not all children with ADHD qualify for IDEA, however, and the eligibility criteria for IDEA vary from state to state. Special education services are most often provided to those children who have significant deficits in the area of academics and/or significant behavioral problems.

If there is a question as to whether a child is eligible, the parents can request that the school conduct an evaluation. The evaluation will usually include a review of records, a teacher observation, and special tests to determine the child's intelligence and academic achievement. If the child qualifies for these services, an individualized education plan is written that will outline the student's abilities; the goals for the student; how progress will be measured; and how the school, student, and parents will work together to meet these goals. Eligible students receive these special education services at no cost to the parents. The students are guaranteed to be in "the least restrictive environment," that is, students should attend classes in the regular classrooms and take part in school activities with children who do not have disabilities. Tutorial services, smaller classrooms, the help of resource teachers in the classroom, untimed tests, and oral testing are all examples of services that can be given under this ruling.

Tutorial Services. Traditional tutorial services are usually the most effective for dealing with academic deficits. Every child's academic needs and learning styles vary. Computerized programs may be helpful, but more significant gains can be made by the one-on-one tutorial help given by a well-trained educational specialist.

Complementary and Alternative Medicine

There is a growing interest in complementary and alternative medicine (CAM) for the treatment of many disorders in pediatric and adult medicine. According to information from the American Academy of Pediatrics, an estimated

20 to 40 percent of healthy children and 50 percent of children with chronic conditions use CAM therapies. The numbers in the adult population are likely much higher. Although there has been some research to evaluate the effectiveness of some CAM treatments, most of the research has been conducted in the adult population.

The American Academy of Pediatrics has emphasized the need for rigorous evaluation of the effectiveness in the use of CAM therapies in children. Many believe that because these therapies are not classified as medication that the therapies are harmless, but this can be far from true. Because CAM treatments are not regulated by the FDA, there is little control over the quality and standardization of these formulations. Also, it is very important to carefully evaluate how any CAM treatments used may interact with standard medications.

Some people have tried using herbs to treat ADHD symptoms. Lemon balm, chamomile, and lavender are said to help with calming and sleep settling and have been used in various herbal remedies to treat the hyperactivity of ADHD. Grape seed extract may help treat inattention, and ginseng and *Gingko biloba* have been said to enhance memory and cognitive performance. However, no well-controlled scientific studies support these claims.

The use of caffeine in treating ADHD children has been addressed in several small studies. Although some positive effects have been demonstrated, anxiety is a common side effect and the positive effects were short lived and failed to match the benefits from central nervous system stimulant medications. Omega-3 fatty acids, which are contained in certain fish oils, collard greens, soy, and walnuts, have been shown in small studies to improve memory skills and concentration in the elderly. At present, however, no scientific studies have shown omega-3 fatty acids to be effective in the treatment of

ADHD. Many other supplements claim to improve the symptoms of ADHD, but none have been shown to be effective.

Further scientific studies of CAM therapies are underway to advance our understanding of the potential positive and negative affects of these treatments. In addition to more research, better regulation of CAM therapies is needed to ensure the safety and consistency of the therapies, should effectiveness be established.

Interactive Metronome Training

Interactive metronome training is a technology that uses a computer to produce a steady reference-beat that individuals must match while they simultaneously perform simple physical exercises. A particular tone is used for each beat. The theory behind this therapy is that the brain improves its capacity for timing and concentration, thus focusing and attention is improved. A small multiple-center study evaluated boys aged six to twelve years with the diagnosis of ADHD. They were assigned to three groups: group 1 received interactive metronome training, group 2 received no intervention, and group 3 received training on selected computer games. The results suggested that the interactive metronome group showed improvements in attention span, motor control, and some academic skills. The study lasted only for several hours, however, and sustained long-term effects have not been proven. Interactive metronome training may be combined with other treatments for ADHD, but no studies have examined the combination of this training with other treatment options. In addition, further studies need to evaluate the long-term outcome of those who receive interactive metronome training once the treatment has been discontinued.

Electroencephalographic Biofeedback

The rationale for biofeedback as a treatment for ADHD comes from the brain imaging and qEEG studies described in chapter 2. When a person is inattentive, slow EEG frequencies occur predominately over the prefrontal and frontal cortex of the brain. As increased awareness and attention is gained, there is an increase in the wave activity. Scientists have found that both laboratory animals and humans can learn to control the production of specific frequencies by monitoring the EEG wave frequency on a screen and learning how to increase concentration and attention.

There has been interest by some in the use of EEG biofeedback as a treatment for ADHD. Joel Lubar at the University of Tennessee studied children with symptoms of inattention and behavioral control issues. He reported that children diagnosed with ADHD demonstrated improved attention and behavioral control after being trained to control the production of EEG activity by concentrating on the wave pattern. Subsequent studies have reported improvement of ADHD symptoms while treatment is ongoing, although there has been some criticism that once the treatment is withdrawn the benefits disappear.

Summary

The treatment of ADHD should be individualized for each patient with a multidisciplinary team organized to address the individual's needs. Although no particular formula exists, there are general guidelines that should be followed to afford optimal treatment. Medication treatment is successful in most children, but other therapies may be necessary to maximize the treatment success. Close monitoring of medication and other therapies is important to track the successes and failures of each intervention. Several new therapies hold promise for the treatment of ADHD, but further research is needed.

5. Creating the Right Environment

"I spent my whole life turning in circles . . . losing things, forgetting about something, and missing out on functions because of my ADD. I want to do whatever I can to help my son have an easier life."
—Statement from a father in an ADHD clinic

It is important to not only have an effective treatment plan for a child with ADHD but also an effective environment that will provide the proper structure and model for the child. In this case, the environment includes the physical space and surroundings, those individuals associated with the child, and their communications and responses to the child.

Designing the Environment

The design of an effective environment should contain the following framework: proper structure of the physical space, clear expectations, proper modeling (demonstration of expected behaviors), strategies available to achieve the expected behaviors, and rewards given when the behavior is achieved. In this chapter, I discuss home, school, and social situations in children and teens to demonstrate how these points can be used to shape the type of behavior desired.

In his book *ADD/ADHD Behavior-Change Resource Kit*, the psychologist Grad L. Flick emphasized that if the wrong information is processed, the wrong outcome is likely. Clear communication of rules and expectations will make a difference in whether a child exhibits positive or negative behavior patterns. The response or consequence to a behavior, whether positive or negative, will also determine whether the behavior occurs again. For example, if there is no consequence for a child who ignored a request to turn off the television and go take a bath one night, the following night he is likely to ignore the request again.

Setting up a proper environment for success for the ADHD individual may be a difficult task. What works in one environment may not generalize to another area of the child's life, and ADHD children do not always learn from their mistakes, so punishing inappropriate behaviors is not always successful. The major focus with the ADHD child should be to develop ways to set the stage for appropriate behaviors.

Home

The most common causes of failure to evoke the desired behaviors in the home environment are poor communication, inappropriate expectations, and lack of consistency. Although certain communication styles may be effective with a child without ADHD, the same style does not always yield the same results in the ADHD child. Children with ADHD frequently do not hear an entire directive because the instructions are cluttered with too much explanation and too many steps. For example, a statement such as, "I want you to go in your room and get ready for school. Be sure to get your homework in your book bag, and don't forget to put your clothes in the clothes basket" gives too much information for the child to assimilate at once. The child likely lost the command after "get ready for school." Instructions should be short, such as "Go to your room, and get dressed for school." Once that task is done, the next command should be "Put your homework in your book bag." Giving only one task to complete at a time increases the likelihood of successful follow-through.

General commands such as "be good" are too broad and do not give clear messages of what behavior is expected. Instructions that will help a child understand expectations should be communicated in a clear, direct fashion: "When we get to the store, hold my hand and stay with me." Another reason that an instruction is not followed is because the parent does not have the child's full attention. Dr. Flick outlined four basic steps of communication in his workbook: get eye contact (make sure the child is looking at you, not the computer screen or television), speak clearly and distinctly in a calm tone of voice, present the command in a simple and concise manner, and verify that the child has heard the command by having him repeat the instructions. If these rules are followed, success in communication will increase.

Psychologist Harvey Parker, founder of Children and Adults with Attention Deficit/Hyperactivity Disorder (CHADD), a nationwide parent support group for ADHD, described the different communication styles that parents use as passive, aggressive, and assertive. Passive communication often puts the directive in the form of a question, "Don't you think it's time to go to bed?" This question sets the stage for a response of "No!" The parent has instantly lost control of the situation. The aggressive communication style is more bullying and critical in its form, "Can't you ever do anything right? I told you to finish that!" Immediately, a negative interaction has been set up between the parent and child. Assertive communication is the best form of communication for parents

Table 5.1 Example of a Chore Chart

	Sun	Mon	Tues	Wed	Thurs	Fri	Sat
Made bed							
Brushed teeth							
Got dressed on time							
Took medicine							
Fed the dog							
Did homework before dinner							
Took dishes to the sink							

and other authority figures to use. An example of an assertive command is, "I need you to pick up your toys so we can get ready for dinner." This communication style is clearly directive, but respectful of the rights and feelings of the child. Because this style also demonstrates to the child good communication skills, a positive model for communication is demonstrated.

Chore lists (Table 5.1) and behavior charts (Table 5.2) can be helpful in making sure that expectations are clearly communicated. The charts should be displayed in an easily viewed area, and they can be modified for use at any age. Repetition of the instructions, new and stimulating ways to encourage the behavior, added color, regular reference to successes, enthusiasm, and frequent and varied rewards will all be helpful in keeping the child with ADHD interested in charting. Choose chores that will improve the child's day-to-day routine. The chores should be easily attainable for the child initially, so that he can be successful and experience the rewards. The recognition that a chore was completed should occur at least daily; for young children several times a day may be needed initially. Once consistent behavior with those particular chores

Table 5.2 Example of a Good Behavior Chart

	Sun	Mon	Tues	Wed	Thurs	Fri	Sat
Used "please" and "thank you"							
Helped my sister with chores							
Said something nice to someone							
Sat quietly in church							
Used good manners at the dinner table							
Shared my toys with my brother							

has been attained, then additional chores can be added or substituted. Behavior charts should have easily reachable goals, which allows the desired behaviors to be rewarded. Each day keep track of the good behaviors, recognize them, and add a star for each time the behavior was exhibited. After a specified number of stars have been earned, a larger reward can be given, such as a getting to watch a special video or going out for pizza. Through these reward systems, the child will become more aware of the desired behaviors.

Success in managing children and teens with ADHD is more likely when there is organization in the home. For some families, this is a difficult task because many parents of ADHD children have ADHD themselves. When the schedule is predictable, however, the household is better organized and the child knows what to expect. Posting a weekly schedule may help a busy family to be better organized.

The pitfall of inappropriate expectations can be avoided through a clear understanding of the developmental level of the child and what should be expected at each level. Many five-year-old children will have difficultly with long periods of sitting quietly. The average attention span of a typical five-year-old is fifteen to twenty minutes and is even less for a five-year-old with ADHD. Expecting them to sit for longer periods is unfair and likely to result in failure. Similarly, an older child with ADHD cannot be expected to complete homework in a chaotic and noisy household, as the distractions will be too extreme. Even when on medication, a child with ADHD may have some fidgety behaviors while sitting and working. To expect a child with ADHD to remain perfectly still is unrealistic, and a small amount of fidgeting should be acceptable as long as it is not interfering with others.

Effective studying is best achieved by having an organized study area that is free of noise and distractions. A comfortable workspace that does not face a window is optimal. Although the kitchen table is often used as a homework spot, it is not the best place for an ADHD child in most cases due to the hustle and bustle of most homes' kitchens. A scheduled time for homework to be completed can be helpful. In addition, allowing the child to take a break every thirty to forty-five minutes can improve concentration and allow for the expenditure of pent up energy.

Scheduling a child with many after-school activities is another bad idea. If a child does not arrive home until the evening, homework must be completed too close to bedtime. This leaves too little time for relaxing and settling down for sleep, which compounds the sleep-settling problems of many children with ADHD. A bedtime routine allowing for some relaxation before the child is expected to fall asleep is important. For younger children this may include reading to the child, story telling, and playing soft music, and for older children playing soft music and pleasure reading for thirty minutes prior to lights out. This routine can be considered a slow decompression for the child. Television watching or playing video games immediately prior to sleep is not recommended because the visual simulation may increase wakefulness in the child.

Messy bedrooms, though common with most children, can be more problematic for a child with ADHD. Because lost and forgotten items are common in the lives of those with ADHD, an effort to keep their bedrooms free of clutter will make the morning routine of getting dressed and out of the house with the proper materials more likely to happen. Some simple tasks will help organize and facilitate the child's daily routine. Require that school clothes are selected the night before, which will speed the dressing process and diminish conflicts. Help to reorganize the child's book bag at least once a week to check for teacher notes and papers that need to be signed and to discard unneeded papers. Ensure that the needed school supplies are available. Post a school assignment sheet for the week in a easily accessed location, which will help to ensure the child is prepared for the next school day. Finally, although this may be difficult in busy families, establishing a predictable schedule at home will help the child stay focused.

Medication in the Home. Forgotten, missed, late, or purposefully not taken medication is a common area of conflict between parents and their children with ADHD. Individuals with ADHD are more likely to forget their medication, however. The child may head to the kitchen to take his medication but then become distracted by a sibling, a pet, the television, or the telephone. Though it is important to teach independence and responsibility, parents of children with ADHD should closely monitor the medication treatment. The medication should be in a safe place, administered one at a time, and carried in a labeled bottle when transported. The majority of medications used to treat ADHD are schedule II drugs, the prescriptions for which require close monitoring by physicians. A lost are stolen prescription can cause significant problems in obtaining refills of the medicine.

Refusal to take the medication or complaints about how the medication makes the child feel should not be ignored. As noted in chapter 4, all of these medications can have adverse side effects. Children are not always able to describe the side effects that they are experiencing, but these may underlie their refusal to take the medication. Although the reluctance or refusal to take the medication may appear as oppositional behavior, appropriate questions about what the child may be feeling will often yield statements such as "it makes me feel sad," "it makes me feel like I don't want to talk to anyone," or "I'm just not hungry when I take the medicine." Certainly, this appetite side effect should be taken seriously. Adjusting mealtimes, encouraging a good breakfast, and allowing late-evening snacks may help with the appetite issue. Once the information is discussed, a call or visit to the prescribing physician for a possible mediation change or dose change can solve the problem in most cases.

Medication refusal also occurs simply because the child does not want to take medication. It may be difficult to swallow or taste bad. Sometimes, a child does not want to do something that others don't have to do. An honest talk with the child about the medication is for and why the medication can help to make things better may be all that is needed. Setting up a behavior chart that includes regularly taking medicine with a reward linked to the accomplished task may be helpful. If medication refusal continues, parents should ask their physician for further suggestions. If a child has decided not to take medication, however, he can figure out how to not take it. Medicines have ended up behind the water fountain, in pants pockets, under the table or bed, or flushed down the toilet. Far more success is achieved when the child agrees to take the medication. A battleground in this area never works well and in the long run may be harmful.

School

Once children enter school, the majority of their waking hours are spent either at the school or involved in extra-curricular activities associated with the school. How much school personnel know about the proper management of ADHD has a great impact on a child's social adjustment, self-esteem, and academic success. Some teachers are very well informed about ADHD and understand accommodations that can make a difference, whereas others are not. Because symptoms of ADHD were not well described until the 1990s, many teachers learned very little about ADHD during their formal education. Although there are resources and workshops available for teachers of children with ADHD, the information is not always accessed. Problems can occur for both the teacher and the child if there is not acceptance and understanding of the disorder.

The development of a partnership between the school personnel and parents to enhance the child's success is of great importance. This section will cover many methods that teachers can use to increase academic successes and decrease the academic agonies for ADHD children, teens, and their teachers. The appendix contains further resources that can be useful for the classroom management of students with ADHD.

Structure in school is needed in both a physical and instructional sense. The classroom arrangement and design can enhance organization and attention. A teacher should make sure the classroom itself is uncluttered and well organized.

Unnecessary material that may serve as a distraction should be removed. The student's work area should be clear and uncluttered. If possible, children with ADHD should be placed near the teacher, in the front row of the classroom, and away from a window to avoid visual distractions. Open classrooms—those with several different centers where students are simultaneously working—are often difficult for children with ADHD to function well in. Lower student-to-teacher ratios are optimal, but not always possible.

To provide a more predictable instructional style, a teacher may:

establish a daily routine with a posted daily schedule;

record assignments in the same place, with ample time to copy the assignments and ask questions;

maintain a master list of all in-class and homework assignments for the students;

have the student maintain a daily assignment book, with a teacher initial to document that the assignment was recorded correctly;

avoid cluttered worksheets;

establish a standard place that homework is to be handed in;

suggest that textbooks be distinguished by different colored book covers;

require a notebook binder with dividers for each subject;

supply a chart or outline to help establish good organization in the note-taking process;

check notebooks periodically to help maintain organization;

set up a regular time each week to clean desks and storage areas; and

prepare the students for a change in routine by explaining the circumstance that caused the change and when it will happen.

To clearly communicate what is expected of an ADHD student in the classroom, a teacher should:

define acceptable and problem behaviors;
make eye contact with the child to be sure there is attention, touching the child's shoulder if necessary;
stand near the child when giving directions;
keep directions short and simple;
repeat directions whenever possible;
display examples of the type of completed work expected;
post the due date of long-term assignments (a monthly calendar may be helpful);
give written instructions when verbal instructions are given; and
stress the importance of a daily review of study materials.

To help ADHD students achieve an increased attention span and better organization skills, a teacher may:

give the student strategies that will help with distractions, such as providing a study carrel;
sit with the child at the front of the auditorium when special functions occur;
suggest that the student use a blank piece of paper as a cover sheet, allowing him to see only the problem that he is currently working on;
teach the student to highlight, underline, or box in important points to help focus on the important facts;
teaching abbreviations to help with the speed of note taking; and
ask the student with restless, fidgety behavior to volunteer for jobs that include motor activity, such as handing out papers or running errands to the school office.

Offering rewards in the classroom to help continue desired behaviors is helpful for children of all ages, although this is most important in the elementary grades. Teachers should reward genuine attempts at a task, not just successes. The rewards might include verbal praise, a small token such as a sticker or a stamp for young children, or an extra classroom privilege for teens. The immediacy of rewards is also important, because delayed rewards or praise may not always reinforce the behavior intended. Teachers who are adept at immediacy of reward will often carry small items in their pockets to use as quick reinforcers. In addition, teachers should praise efforts at independence and problem solving. This point is especially important for a child who has low self-esteem. The attention given to the effort may be all that is needed to bolster the student's confidence and encourage further efforts in achievement.

For the child with ADHD, modifications may be needed to allow for successes in the classroom, such as devising a 504 Plan or seeking special education programs, as discussed in chapter 4. Some commonly employed methods to help ADHD children with classroom success include:

dividing class work into smaller segments;
handing out worksheets one at a time to diminish the feelings of being overwhelmed;
allowing the use of a laptop for classroom work or note taking;
allowing the use of a tape recorder;
developing a secret code, such as a shoulder tap, to remind the student to get back on task if he is daydreaming, while avoiding embarrassment;
giving the child a written copy of homework assignments, even if the assignment is written on the board;

keeping the child abreast of missing assignments and
   allowing the opportunity to make them up; and
pairing the student with an organized, non-ADHD child
   when group assignments are given.

The Social World

Navigating the social world can be difficult at times for
anyone, although individuals with ADHD may have particular problems. Self-esteem is partially determined by how one
is viewed by others, and peer acceptance and relationships are
especially important for children and teens. Individuals with
ADHD do not tend to have problems making friends, although
they sometimes have problems keeping friends. Children with
ADHD are often accused of acting younger than they are.
Those diagnosed with ADHD CT and ADHD-HI have poor
listening skills, impulsiveness, disruptive and fidgety behavior,
and hyperactivity. These behaviors make following instructions and rules during games, sharing, playing cooperatively,
and even participating in a conversation difficult.

The majority of the complaints center around behavioral
issues that occur in social situations. At times, some individuals with ADHD will seem to function without a filter in their
brain. Whatever thought enters their minds comes straight
out of their mouths. This social ineptness is likely due to the
decreased level of activity in the prefrontal and frontal cortex
of the brain, as discussed in chapter 2. The executive functions that occur in this region of the brain relate to planning,
initiating, problem solving, inhibition of impulsivity, and
understanding of the behavior of others. All of these functions are very important for appropriate social interaction to
occur.

In his book *ADHD and the Nature of Self-Control*, Russell Barkley noted the difficulties of behavioral inhibition. Although theoretical, his ideas offer an excellent explanation as to why those with ADHD have such difficulty in social situations. According to Barkley, there are several problems that contribute to this lack of behavioral inhibition. First, individuals with ADHD have a poor working memory (inability to hold events in mind), poor hindsight, poor forethought, limited self-awareness, a diminished sense of time, and delayed time organization. Second, they show a delayed internalization of speech. This lack of internalization causes the individual to have a decreased ability to reflect on a situation, poor self-questioning and problem solving, poor ability to follow instructions, and delayed moral reasoning. The third major factor is an immature self-regulation of mood, motivation, and arousal, meaning that individuals with ADHD have less of an ability to be self-motivated and self-directed to complete tasks. They may experience mood swings, and there may be inconsistent performance. The final major contributor to poor behavioral self-regulation is a limited ability to take the information available and synthesize it into a reasonable working response or action.

Although medication can be very helpful in the child's social adjustment and performance, for some individuals, proper planning and selection of social situations is often necessary. Large group activities, functions without clearly set rules and limits, and poorly supervised situations all can result in a negative outcome for the ADHD child. For instance, being in a large group makes it more difficult for the person with ADHD to listen to what is being said by those around him, and misinterpretation can lead to a conflict. Impulsive aggressive behaviors are not unusual in situations such as this. The push, shove, or negative words can cause peers to view the child as someone to avoid.

A talented athlete with ADHD may be tagged as a poor team member due to an inability to pay attention to the coach or what is going on the field. Impulsive or unplanned aggression from a child with ADHD is not unusual in a sports situation, when adrenaline is running high. A tackle on the soccer field or a slammed racket on the tennis court may happen, even though the child understands that this is wrong. In such situations, the child may be too overwhelmed by external stimulation to be thinking clearly about appropriate behavior. The consequences of the behaviors such as these include team penalties, lost games, and angry teammates.

As a child grows older, poor behavioral inhibition becomes even more problematic. For example, teens with inadequately treated ADHD are more likely to develop substance abuse disorders. Tobacco, alcohol, and other illicit drug use begins earlier and lasts longer in individuals with ADHD. Teens with ADHD have a higher incidence of motor vehicle accidents, speeding violations, driving while intoxicated, and license suspensions. These teens may be technically good drivers, but are oblivious to the speed limit, the curve in the road, or the approaching car. Cell phones, adjusting the radio, or talking to friends are all distracters for teen drivers with ADHD.

Adjusting the Environment

The first step in helping a child or teen navigate successfully in social situations is to anticipate those situations that will cause problems. Such situations may then be avoided or at least adjusted to lessen the chance of problems arising. Proper expectations for each situation should be very clearly discussed with the child shortly before the planned function, as should the consequences if negative behaviors arise. By going through this routine with each situation, the child with ADHD will be able to learn how to approach social situations appropriately, and self-esteem will improve with each success.

Elementary-Age Children and Preteens

When a child has difficulty participating in team sports, consider encouraging sports such as swim team, track, karate, tennis, or golf. If a child enjoys team sports like baseball, keep in mind that a position that requires a higher activity level such as pitcher or catcher will likely hold the child's attention better than a position in the outfield, which may end up with more flowers picked than balls caught.

If large parties or gatherings are more stimulating than the child can handle, plan smaller group settings that are well supervised. The more organized the function is and the less free-play that occurs, the better things will go.

When a child has difficulty making and keeping friends, plan one-on-one outings that will give more structure such as going out to a movie or for pizza. Until social skills are well developed, it is best to avoid having more than one guest at a time. Prior to the outing, remind the child of proper manners and expectations.

When a child is prone to disruptive and impulsive behaviors on a shopping trip or at a restaurant, give clear guidelines of the rules and expectations for the outing. If the child falters, a warning should be communicated clearly, while making sure to have the child's full attention. If the warning is not heeded, there should an abrupt end to the outing.

Learn to recognize those times of the day when problem behaviors are more likely to occur, such as when medication wears off or with fatigue or hunger. If possible, plan functions to avoid these "bewitching times." If there does seem to be a regular pattern to the time of day that trouble occurs, consult the physician to be sure that medication dose and timing is correct.

Teens

As teens get older, the hyperactivity is often replaced with feelings of restlessness. Therefore, long periods of unstructured time may increase dissatisfaction and risky behavior. Helping the teen focus his energies into fruitful, fun, and productive behaviors will improve self-esteem and increase social awareness. Discuss the teen's interests and skills, and encourage him to further develop a hobby or skill. On holidays and during the summer, involve teens in volunteer work and planned activities with family or friends or suggest they get a part-time job.

Help teens to remember others. Problems with behavioral inhibition result in difficulties with delayed gratification. This often means that the teen with ADHD will put his needs before others. Work on the self-centered behaviors by reminding him of important dates, planning to help others, and modeling the appropriate caring behaviors.

Provide supervision during potential risk-taking activities, such as boating, water or snow skiing, dirt biking, or hunting. Teens in general will "live for the day" and assume that they are invincible, and such behavior is magnified in the ADHD teens due to their impulsivity. If the situation seems too dangerous, then don't let it happen. It is important to have fixed rules of safety that must be followed when dealing with ADHD teens, such as the requirement that a helmet or life-vest be worn. If the rules are not followed, then the activity should not be allowed to continue.

Because teens with ADHD tend to seek out those with like characteristics, they may be associating with others with high-risk behaviors. Insist on meeting your child's friends, and, if possible, talk with their parents as well to learn what amount of supervision they are giving. Let the teen know that you will check to be sure of the details.

In her book *Teenagers with ADD: A Parents' Guide*, Chris Zeigler Dendy suggested that when teens are having problems making and keeping friends, the parents should invite his friends on outings, provide tips on relating to friends, help critique problem areas, and find teachable moments to give examples of a better way to act. For example, if a teen complains that no one likes him, use that as an opening to say, "I could give you some tips so making friends might be easier." That may open the door to suggestions such as how to be a good listener or the importance of not monopolizing conversations.

The majority of individuals with ADHD have normal intelligence and no other behavioral problems or learning disorders. However, there are times that simple suggestions are not enough. Formal therapy with a professional who is well versed in social skills training can help a struggling teen to become more adept at approaching social situations. This therapy is best achieved through group practice with peers. Acting out certain social situations with a critique from the therapist will help the teen understand appropriate ways to approach different social situations. Short-term therapy may prevent long-term problems with self-esteem, improve mood and social adjustment, and even improve academic performance.

Summary

Creating an environment that provides the proper structure and model for those with ADHD is a key factor in the overall success of their daily lives. Design of the right environment requires appropriate arrangement of the physical space, clearly stated expectations, and recognition of successes as they occur so that the desired behaviors are reinforced. Although the home, school, and social environments all need similar designs, the differences in these varied surroundings must be taken into account. Avoiding the most common pitfalls, including poor communication, inappropriate expectations, and lack of consistency, will ensure a more positive outcome for individuals with ADHD.

6. Searching for a Cure

"I just want to be normal, like everybody else. Will that ever happen?"
— Timothy, fifteen-year-old, at a follow-up visit

Research in ADHD has exploded in the last several years, but many questions about the disorder remain unanswered. For instance, why do various treatments work for some, but not others? Is there a way to tell which individuals will respond best to the different treatments? Are there diagnostic tests for ADHD available that can make the diagnosis with certainty? Can ADHD be prevented? What are the best approaches to finding a cure?

Medical and psychological research can be divided into two major groups, clinical trials and basic research. Clinical trials use human volunteers to study the safety, effectiveness, and side effects of medications and possible long-term problems with certain treatments. Interventional clinical trials evaluate experimental and new treatments for disorders or new ways of using already-known therapies used in the treatment of other disorders or in other groups of individuals. Observational clinical trials evaluate the impact of different health issues in large groups of people in their natural settings, such as evaluating the differences in the rate of ADHD in each state. Basic research investigates the anatomy and physiology of those with particular disorders. Because there is growing evidence that ADHD is largely caused by genetic factors, basic research in this area often involves looking for the genes that control particular functions in the body as well as mutations in those genes. This type of research also examines the neurochemistry, neuroanatomy, and nerve pathways of individuals with ADHD compared to those who do not have the disorder.

Funding for clinical and basic research comes from many different sources, including medical institutions, pharmaceutical companies, private foundations, and voluntary groups, such as physicians and psychologists in private practice who are interested in conducting research. Federal agencies such as the National Institutes of Health and its subsidiary, the National Institute of Mental Health; the Department of Defense; and the Department of Veteran's Affairs all fund many projects. The research may take place either at a single site or as a multiple-center project.

Clinical Trials

The National Institutes of Health has developed a website (www.ClinicalTrials.gov) for those interested in participating in a clinical trial. This site has excellent general information on clinical trials and summarizes the trials that are looking for volunteers. There are guidelines in each study of who can participate (inclusion criteria) and those who cannot participate (exclusion criteria). For example, some studies may want only people who have been diagnosed with a particular disorder, only males, or only those who are a certain age, which are inclusion criteria. Exclusion criteria may not allow someone to participate who is taking medication, is younger than requested, or has other health problems.

Each clinical trial is required to obtain a written informed consent from the volunteers. This consent contains information about the clinical trial, with details such as the purpose of the study, how long it will last, what is required of the volunteer, and who are the contacts to call if there is a problem.

There is also information about the possible benefits and risks for the participant. Possible risks of the research may include side effects of the experimental treatment, ineffective treatment, or doctor visits or hospital stays due to complications from the treatments. All known potential risks must be outlined in the consent form.

The study plan for each clinical trial is called a protocol. The protocol describes the research questions to be answered, type of people who can participate, procedures, medications, and length of the study. The protocol also outlines the schedule of the study and how the participants will be monitored. Every clinical trial must be approved by an institutional review board, and federal law requires that every institution that conducts or supports research on human participants have an institutional review board. This board is a committee of physicians, statisticians, researchers, community advocates, and others who are appointed to ensure that the trial is ethical and that the rights and safety of the participants are protected. The board initially approves of the project and it periodically reviews the ongoing research for any problems or potential violations of the protocol.

Clinical trials are typically divided in to five major categories: (1) prevention trials, which investigate ways to prevent disease; (2) diagnostic trials, which look for better tests for the diagnosis of particular diseases or disorders; (3) screening trials, which evaluate better ways to detect certain disorders; (4) treatment trials, which test new treatments or a new combination of treatments; and (5) quality-of-life trials, which search for ways to improve the life and comfort level of those with a disease or disorder.

Clinical trials typically occur in four phases. Phase I trials test an experimental treatment in a small group of eighty or fewer people for the fist time to evaluate its safely, investigate the effective dose range, and identify side effects. Phase II trials evaluate a larger group of people (up to 300) looking at the same issues. Phase III trials examine outcomes in much larger groups (up to 3000) to confirm the effectiveness of the treatment, further evaluate side effects, and compare it to other treatments for the same disorder. Finally, phase IV trials occur after the FDA or other authorities have released the treatment for use, when further information is sought concerning side effects, any newly discovered potential risks and benefits, and best way to use the treatment.

Brain Imaging Trials

As discussed in chapter 2, brain imaging studies have shown structural differences in several different areas of the brain in individuals with ADHD as compared to those without the disorder. The reported differences are minor, however. In addition, the studies examined only a small number of individuals and the results across similar studies have not always been consistent.

A phase II observational study is being conducted at the University Medical Center in Utrecht to determine if the brain differences found in ADHD children and teens are due to a disruption in brain development or a delay in development. This study is using diffusion tensor imaging (DT-MRI), which is more sensitive than previous MRIs for evaluating brain development. By using DT-MRI, a researcher is able to look at the white matter of the brain, which consists of billions of insulated nerve fibers that carry messages to and from the cerebral cortex. This trial includes 300 children and teens and will help to determine whether consistent changes occur at particular ages or in particular individuals who have ADHD.

The National Institute of Mental Health is conducting a DT-MRI trial entitled "Anatomic MRI Brain Imaging of White Matter in Children." The participants are identical twins in which one twin has ADHD and the other does not. The purpose of this study is to look at certain areas of these genetically identical twins to determine if there are differences in the twins' brain structure and size, which may lead to new information about the environmental effects on brain anatomy in individuals with ADHD.

Genetic Studies

The current school of thought is that ADHD is a complex disorder and that mutations in several genes are involved in its development. Although twin studies and family histories have shown that ADHD may be inherited from one generation to the next, there are still no consistently identified genetic markers that will absolutely make the diagnosis of ADHD.

The National Human Genome Research Institute is conducting the "Genetic Analysis of Attention Deficit Hyperactivity Disorder" study to determine if a biochemical marker (a chemical or substance in the brain tissue) exists that may correlate with genetic markers for ADHD. The study includes 4000 individuals in two groups: the Paisa, an isolated population in Colombia, and the members of U.S. families that have a child with ADHD. This study will use a new scanning technique, proton magnetic resonance spectroscopy, which measures the concentrations of different chemical components within brain tissues, to compare the prefrontal regions of individuals with or without ADHD.

The National Institute of Environmental Health Sciences is sponsoring another observational study on the genetics of

ADHD, entitled "Measurement of Cytogenetic Endpoints in Lymphocytes of Children Diagnosed with ADHD and Treated with Methylphenidate or Adderall." This study will be conducted at Duke University in North Carolina. A previous study showed that taking methylphenidate for ADHD may result in changes to the genetic material in blood cells (lymphocytes). The changes did not appear to be directly linked to an increased risk of disease or other problems, but only a small number of children were included in the previous study, and all of them lived in South Texas near oil refineries. This new study will further investigate if damage occurs to genetic material with long-term methylphenidate treatment in children with ADHD.

Nutritional Studies

In recent years, several nutritional deficiencies have been described in children with ADHD. Small studies have suggested that supplements with magnesium, calcium, and essential fatty acids may improve attention span and cognition. In addition, anecdotal evidence suggests that if the amount of carbohydrate is decreased in an ADHD child's diet and protein is increased, behavior and concentration improves. Researchers at Children's Hospital of Philadelphia are evaluating the diets of children with and without ADHD. The study will assess the protein, carbohydrate, fat, calorie, and specific nutrient intake. This is a prospective study, one that evaluates events as they happen, and will record the natural dietary habits of the children.

Interventional Studies

Interventional trials evaluate the effectiveness of new treatments or a new combination of treatments. There are many such studies in the area of ADHD, and a few of these are described in this section. Several issues must be taken into account when novel treatments are evaluated. To prevent bias in the study population—for instance, comparing one study group that has only boys to another group with both genders—the trial should evaluate a random sample of individuals. This minimizes the differences among groups by having those with different characteristics evenly distributed throughout the study groups. Another way to avoid bias is to blind the participant as to the treatment received, that is, the participant would not know if he is getting the real drug or a placebo. A double-blind study is one in which neither the participant nor the study staff measuring the outcomes know who is receiving the experimental drug and who is receiving a placebo; only a researcher who is not actually involved in the measurements has this information. In a crossover study, a participant is placed on the active treatment for one period and then, after a rest period, is placed on the placebo or vice versa. This way each participant's response can be evaluated while on placebo and on the experimental drug.

NRP104. This is a new form of an old stimulant that is being studied to be used in the treatment of ADHD. NRP104 (lisdexamfetamine dimesylate) is an amphetamine joined to a specific amino acid, which is a building block of proteins. This amino acid inactivates the drug, which only becomes active when a chemical reaction occurs in the body that snips off the amino acid. The drug is converted to its active state at a fixed and steady rate over the course of the day. For those active drugs with an abuse potential, the fixed rate of conversion might make the substances less appealing if there is no notable "high." NRP104 is intended to provide better overdose protection and to reduce the potential for addiction or misuse compared to currently available amphetamines, while providing effective treatment of ADHD.

In a phase II classroom trial of NRP104, investigators established the most effective dose of Adderall XR by studying fifty children aged six to twelve years during a three-week period. For one-week periods, in a cross-over design for a total of three weeks, participants received NRP104 at a dose approximately equivalent to the child's most effective Adderall XR dose, Adderall XR at the child's most effective dose, or a placebo. The results demonstrated consistently improved classroom behavior and functioning when the children received either NRP104 or Adderall XR as compared to placebo. Adverse events reported by the participants were mild to moderate. The most common adverse side effects for NRP104 were difficulty falling asleep (8 percent), decreased appetite (6 percent), and poor sleep (4 percent), and those for Adderall XR were decreased appetite (4 percent), abdominal pain (4 percent), difficulty falling asleep (2 percent), and vomiting (2 percent).

There is an ongoing phase III study that is designed to evaluate the safety and effectiveness of NRP104 in treating adults eighteen to fifty-five years of age diagnosed with moderate to severe ADHD. This is a multiple-center study sponsored by New River Pharmaceuticals, the manufacturer NRP104.

ABT-089. The new drug ABT-089 has been developed to act at the nicotinic receptor sites in the brain. Nicotinic receptors play a role in complex brain functions such as attention, memory, and processing information. These receptors seem to be most important in the presynaptic areas of the nerve endings (Fig. 6.1). Research has shown that these nicotinic receptors are involved in disorders such as Alzheimer's and Parkinson's diseases, Tourette's syndrome, schizophrenia,

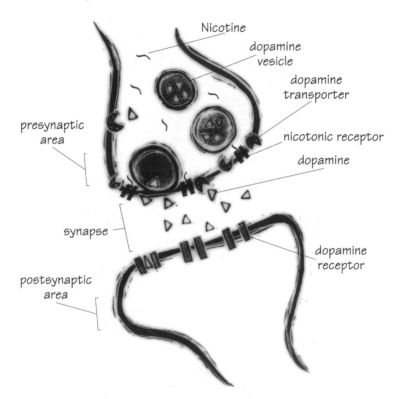

Figure 6.1. When nicotine is present at the nicotinic receptor site, dopamine is more rapidly released, thus increasing the amount of dopamine in the synapse.

depression, and ADHD. By binding to these receptors, nicotine appears to promote the release of dopamine in the presynaptic area, thus increasing the amount of dopamine in the synapse. This action is similar to the stimulant medications that have been used to treat ADHD. This fact may be why a higher percentage of ADHD individuals smoke cigarettes as compared to the general population (40 percent versus 26 percent). A 1996 study of adults with ADHD found that when nicotine patches were applied their symptoms improved. With nicotine use, however, there are potential cardiac side effects and addiction issues that can occur. Researchers at Massachusetts General in Boston completed a small study to evaluate the effectiveness of ABT-089 in treating the symptoms of ADHD, and they reported improved memory and concentration in the individuals who used ABT-089. A multiple-center, phase II study is planned to further evaluate this drug's effectiveness.

Herbal Treatments. Although many herbal remedies have been proposed for use in the treatment of ADHD (see chapter 4), little scientific research has been conducted in this area. Two studies that appear to be well designed are evaluating proposed herbal treatments for ADHD.

Wendy Weber at Bastyr University in Seattle is conducting an interventional, phase II study to evaluate the effectiveness of St. John's wort (*Hypericum perforatum*) in the treatment of ADHD. St. John's wort is a plant that has been shown to have some effect on levels of serotonin, one of the neurotransmitters affected in individuals with depression. The participants will get either the herbal product or a placebo three times a day and will have their symptoms of ADHD evaluated on a weekly basis and the side effects assessed.

Another herbal study is being conducted at the Canadian Center for Functional Medicine in British Columbia. It will evaluate the effectiveness of L-theanine, an amino acid found in green tea, in the treatment of ADHD. This phase II trial will evaluate 100 boys with ADHD for the effects of L-theanine on behavior, cognitive performance, and sleep quality.

Aripiprazole (Abilify). As discussed in chapter 4, some individuals with ADHD do not respond to stimulant medication. Abilify is a new antipsychotic medication that is approved for use in the treatment of bipolar disorder and schizophrenia in adults. The mode of action of Abilify is related to a stabilization of dopamine and serotonin transmission. This drug appears to improve the function of dopamine and serotonin receptors, thus enhancing transmission of nerve signals in the brain. The New York State Psychiatric Institute is conducting a phase II study to evaluate the use of Abilify as a combination medication in the treatment of ADHD. Abilify will be added to the stimulant medication (either Adderall XR or Concerta) in those who do not or only partially respond to stimulant treatment and their outcomes will be evaluated.

Cognitive Behavioral Therapy. Recent evidence suggests that more than 50 percent of those diagnosed with ADHD as children will continue to have problematic symptoms throughout adulthood, and up to 5 percent of adults in the United States may have the disorder. Adults with ADHD often have increased problems with occupational underachievement, relationship problems, and an overall reduced quality of life. An interventional study sponsored by the National Institute of Mental Health and conducted at Massachusetts General Hospital will investigate whether cognitive behavioral therapy is more effective than ADHD education and relaxation techniques in treating adults with ADHD.

Treating ADHD in Children with Comorbidities

Comorbid is the term used to describe two conditions that occur together. Many disorders coexist with ADHD, including learning disabilities, mood disorders, behavioral disorders, and other health issues. The following studies are a few of the research projects evaluating ADHD and comorbid disorders.

Epilepsy. One-third of children with epilepsy also have ADHD. Although stimulant medication is a very effective treatment in the management of ADHD, there are long-standing

concerns that the stimulants might affect the seizure frequency of those with coexisting epilepsy. A cross-over study is
being conducted at the Harvard Medical School to evaluate
the safety and effectiveness of Concerta (a long-acting
methylphenidate) in the treatment of children with both
ADHD and epilepsy.

Oppositional Defiant Disorder. Many children with
ADHD also have been diagnosed with oppositional defiant
disorder. A study is being conducted to assess the effectiveness and safety of SPD503 (guanfacine hydrochloride) in
the treatment of children ages six to twelve years with both
ADHD and oppositional behaviors. SPD503 has been
shown to be an effective treatment for ADHD. Due to the
action on the prefrontal cortex of the brain, it is thought
that this substance may modulate oppositional behavior as
well. This study is a phase III multiple-center study sponsored
by Shire Pharmaceuticals and is in the beginning stages of
investigation.

Substance Abuse. There is an increased incidence of substance abuse in those with ADHD. The outcome of teens
and adults treated for substance abuse who also have ADHD
is poor, and the risk of persistent behavior problems is higher
in those ADHD individuals who abuse drugs and alcohol.
Research has shown that the majority of those with ADHD
who are in treatment for substance abuse are not treated for
their ADHD.

The National Institute on Drug Abuse is sponsoring two
studies to evaluate whether medication therapy for ADHD
will improve the treatment for substance abuse. The first
study will compare the use of Concerta to a placebo treatment
in adolescents aged thirteen to eighteen years. Three hundred
participants will be recruited at eleven different sites. All of
the participants will also receive cognitive-behavioral therapy

as the standard treatment for the substance abuse. The other study will evaluate medication use in the treatment of adults who have both ADHD and marijuana dependence. Atomoxetine, a medication approved for the treatment of ADHD, with be combined with motivational therapy to determine if the combined therapy will reduce the use of marijuana in those individuals.

Bipolar Disorder. A Brazilian study is investigating the use of aripiprazole (Abilify) in the treatment of children with bipolar disorder and ADHD. As noted above, Abilify stabilizes dopamine and serotonin transmission in the brain, which may help to treat the overlapping symptoms of ADHD and bipolar disorder. The study will investigate whether aripiprazole reduces mania scores compared to placebo, significantly reduces ADHD behavioral scores compared to placebo, without a significant weight gain, which is a major issue for some of the other antipsychotics that have been used in the treatment of bipolar disorder.

Basic Research

Most treatments have their origins in basic research, although many questions about ADHD remain. Additional research is needed to better understand the development of attention, motivation, and other higher executive functions across the life span. Factors that present a risk of developing ADHD or protection from the disorder need to be investigated further. A better understanding of the neurobiological differences across the different subtypes of ADHD will help with treatment of the diverse individuals who share this disorder. Brain imaging studies are providing new information about the basic neural circuits involved in ADHD. Treatments for the cognitive and behavioral deficits seen in ADHD can be improved through the development of animal models, using rats, mice, and monkeys to test new treatments for this disorder. In addition, there are still no cognitive tests for the diagnosis of the core symptoms of ADHD. The development of such a tool will help expedite the treatment of those with the disorder. Below are a few of the basic research studies that have implications for future work in the area of ADHD.

The Effect of Methylphenidate on Genes

A common treatment for ADHD is the stimulant methylphenidate. As noted earlier in this chapter, a recent study reported possible genetic changes in certain blood cells of children who had been treated with this drug. Although the study protocol had some problems, concern was raised about the potential of genetic toxicity with the use of methylphenidate. Swiss researchers evaluated the changes in the genetic material in cultured human blood cells (lymphocytes) exposed to methylphenidate. High concentrations of methylphenidate did not induce either structural or numerical changes in the chromosomes within the cells. Another methylphenidate study was performed on mice to evaluate genetic changes. A dose over 200 times that used in humans for the treatment of ADHD was used, and no noted genetic changes were found in the bone marrow cells of the mice.

Brain Changes

Dopamine and norepinephrine levels affect a person's ability to pay attention and concentrate. Differences in several areas of the brain are found in those with ADHD, for instance, these individuals tend to have a smaller cerebellar area, especially the back and lower portions, the cerebellar vermis (see chapter 2 for more details). The pathway for dopamine activity in this area of the cerebellum is not clearly understood. Researchers at the University of Kentucky studied tissue from the cerebellar area of rats and monkeys to investigate dopamine or norepinephrine pathways in this part of the brain. They found that norepinephrine levels were significantly higher than dopamine levels in the cerebellar vermis. Thus, in individuals with ADHD whose cerebellar vermis is small, norepinephrine may play a larger role. This fact may highlight why there is variability in the response to different medications in those with ADHD.

A study conducted on monkeys at the Yale University School of Medicine found that blocking the receptors that help to transport norepinephrine and dopamine through the synapses in the prefrontal cortex created the symptoms of ADHD. The animals showed impaired working memory, increased impulsivity, and hyperactivity. This study lends further evidence to the idea that abnormalities or diminished function in the prefrontal cortex occur in at least some individuals with ADHD.

Summary

Questions regarding the causes of ADHD and ways to diagnose and better treat the disorder are being investigated through the research of many dedicated individuals. Continued evaluation of the safety and effectiveness of the present treatments and long-term outcome of those who have used the various treatments require well-designed clinical studies.

Researchers are working to identify the genetic markers and the other possible causes of ADHD and to find a way, if there is one, to prevent the disorder from developing in those with a predisposition for ADHD. Ultimately, researchers are searching not only for excellent and safe treatments for ADHD, but also a real cure.

Appendix:
Additional Resources

This appendix contains the contact information for general resources and support and advocacy groups, web sites, and recommended reading that will provide additional information for parents, teachers, and others who are interested in the management and treatment for ADHD.

General Resources

American Academy of Child and Adolescent Psychiatry
3615 Wisconsin Avenue NW
Washington, DC 20016-3007
Tel. (202) 966-7300
www.aacap.org

American Academy of Pediatrics
National Headquarters
141 Northwest Point Blvd.
Elk Grove Village, IL 60007-1098
Tel. (847) 434-4000
www.aap.org

American Psychological Association
750 First Street NE
Washington, DC 20002-4242
Tel. (202) 336-5500 or (800) 374-2721
www.apa.org

Attention Deficit Disorder Association
15000 Commerce Parkway, Suite C
Mount Laurel, NJ 08054
Tel. (856) 439-9099
www.add.org

Learning Disabilities Association of America
4156 Library Road, Pittsburgh, PA 15234-1349
Tel. (412) 341-1515
www.ldanatl.org

National Alliance on Mental Illness
Colonial Place Three
2107 Wilson Blvd., Suite 300
Arlington, VA 22201-3042
Tel. (703) 524-7600 or (800) 950-6264
www.nami.org

National Center for Learning Disabilities
381 Park Avenue S, Suite 1401
New York, NY 10016
Tel. (212) 545-7510 or (888) 575-7373
www.ncld.org

National Dissemination Center for Children with Disabilities
P.O. Box 1492
Washington, DC 20013
Tel. (800) 695-0285
www.nichcy.org

National Institute of Mental Health
Public Information and Communications Branch
6001 Executive Blvd., Room 8184, MSC 9663
Bethesda, MD 20892-9663
Tel. (301) 443-4513 or (866) 615-6464
www.nimh.nih.gov

U.S. Department of Health and Human Services
Substance Abuse and Mental Health Administration
Center for Mental Health Services
PO Box 42557 Washington, DC 20015
Tel. (800) 789-2647
www.mentalhealth.samhsa.gov/cmhs

Parent Support and Advocacy

Children and Adults with Attention Deficit/Hyperactivity
Disorder
8181 Professional Place, Suite 150
Landover, MD 20785
Tel. (301) 306-7070
www.chadd.org

Council for Exceptional Children
1110 North Glebe Road, Suite 300
Arlington, VA 22201
Tel. (703) 620-3660
www.ideapractices.org

National Association of Protection and Advocacy Systems
900 Second Street NE, Suite 211
Washington, DC 20002
Tel. (202) 408-9514

National Resource Center on ADHD
Children and Adults with Attention Deficit/Hyperactivity
Disorder
8181 Professional Place, Suite 150
Landover, MD 20785
Tel. (800) 233-4050
www.help4adhd.org

Parent Advocacy Coalition for Educational Rights
8161 Normandale Blvd., Minneapolis, MN 55437
Tel. (952) 838-9000
www.pacer.org

Publication Resources

ADD Warehouse
300 NW 70th Avenue, Suite 102
Plantation, FL 33317
Tel. (954) 792-8100 or (800) 233-9273
www.addwarehouse.com

Attention Deficit Disorder Resources
223 Tacoma Avenue S, Suite 100
Tacoma, WA 98402
Tel. (253) 759-5085
www.addresources.org

Education Resources

Office of Special Education and Rehabilitative Services
U.S. Department of Education
400 Maryland Avenue SW
Washington, DC 20202-7100
Tel. (202) 245-7468
www.ed.gov/about/offices/list/osers/index.html

U.S. Department of Education
400 Maryland Avenue SW
Washington, DC 20202
Tel. (800) 872-5327
www.ed.gov
www.ed.gov/teachers

Web Sites

www.advocacyinstitute.org

The Advocacy Institute is a nonprofit organization dedicated to the development of products, projects, and services that work to improve the lives of people with disabilities. The Advocacy Institute provides consultative services to educators, counselors, service providers, parents, students, organizations, government entities, and others.

www.cdc.gov

The Centers for Disease Control and Prevention is one of the thirteen major operating components of the U.S. Department of Health and Human Services. Their web site may be searched for ADHD-related conferences and workshops, resources, and publications, as well as updates about ongoing ADHD research projects.

www.childdevelopmentinfo.com

The Child Development Institute web site provides information on child development, child psychology, parenting, learning, health, and safety, as well as childhood disorders such as ADHD, dyslexia, and autism. Comprehensive resources and practical suggestions for parents covering toddlers to teens are available.

www.osepideasthatwork.org

This web site provides easy access to information from research to practice initiatives funded by the U.S. Office of Special Education Programs that address the provisions of the Individual with Disabilities Education Act and the No Child Left Behind Act.

www.wrightslaw.com
Wrightslaw's web site provides information about special education law, education law, and advocacy for children with disabilities. Free resources on dozens of topics, such as Individual with Disabilities Education Act, special education, advocacy, training, and seminars are available.

Suggested Reading

Books

Barkley, Russell A. 2000. *Taking Charge of ADHD: The Complete, Authoritative Guide for Parents.* Rev. ed. Guilford Press, New York, 321 pp.

Batshaw, Mark L., ed. 2002. *Children with Disabilities.* Paul H. Brookes Publishing Co., Baltimore, Md., 870 pp.

Bloomquist, Michael L. 2006. *Skills Training for Children with Behavior Problems: A Parent and Practitioner Guidebook.* Rev. ed. Guilford Press, New York, 242 pp.

Flick, Grad L. 1998. *ADD/ADHD Behavior-Change Resource Kit: Ready-to-Use Strategies and Activities for Helping Children with Attention Deficit Hyperactivity Disorder.* Center for Applied Research in Education, West Nyack, N.Y., 391 pp.

Hallowell, Edward M., and John J. Ratey. 2006. *Delivered from Distraction: Getting the Most out of Life with Attention Deficit Disorder.* Ballantine, New York, 379 pp.

Parker, Harvey C. 1992. *The ADD Hyperactivity Handbook for Schools: Effective Strategies for Identifying and Teaching Students with Attention Deficit Hyperactivity Disorders in Elementary and Secondary Schools.* Specialty Press, Plantation, Fla., 330 pp.

Parker, Harvey C. 1994. *The ADD Hyperactivity Workbook for Parents, Teachers, and Kids.* Specialty Press, Plantation, Fla., 142 pp.

Reiff, Michael I. 2004. *ADHD: A Complete and Authoritative Guide for Parents.* American Academy of Pediatrics, Elk Grove Village, Ill., 354 pp.

Wodrich, David L., and Ara J. Schmitt. 2006. *Patterns of Learning Disorders: Working Systematically from Assessment to Intervention.* Guilford Press, New York, 306 pp.

Zeigler Dendy, Chris A. 1995. *Teenagers with ADD: A Parents' Guide.* Woodbine House, Bethesda, Md., 370 pp.

Magazines and Newsletters

ADDitude Magazine
Tel. (888) 762-8475
www.additudemag.com
The ADHD Report by Russell A. Barkley, Ph.D.
Tel. (800) 365-7006
www.guilford.com

Attention! Magazine
Bimonthly publication for members of Children and Adults with Attention Deficit Hyperactivity Disorder
Tel. (301) 306-7070
www.chadd.org

Exceptional Parent
Tel. (201) 489-4111
www.eparent.com

The New CHADD Information and Resource Guide to AD/HD
Benefit of membership in Children and Adults with Attention Deficit Hyperactivity Disorder
Tel. (800) 233-4050
www.chadd.org

Index

Understanding Health and Sickness Series
Miriam Bloom, Ph.D., General Editor

Also in this series